The 17 Day Diet
COOKBOOK

80 All New Recipes for Healthy Weight Loss

DR MIKE MORENO

SIMON & SCHUSTER

London · New York · Sydney · Toronto · New Delhi

A CBS COMPANY

D0452752

First published in Great Britain by Simon & Schuster UK Ltd, 2012
A CBS COMPANY

Text copyright © 2012 by 17 Day Diet, Inc.
Photographs copyright © 2012 by Nisha Sondhe

Simon & Schuster UK Ltd
1st Floor
222 Gray's Inn Road
London
WC1X 8HB

www.simonandschuster.co.uk

Simon & Schuster Australia, Sydney
Simon & Schuster India, New Delhi

A CIP catalogue record for this book
is available from the British Library.

ISBN: 978-1-84983-925-9

Printed and bound in Italy by
by L.E.G.O. SpA

*This book is dedicated to the millions of people who are following
the 17 Day Diet to get in shape, reclaim their health
and change their lifestyle for the better.*

ACKNOWLEDGEMENTS

As a family doctor, my passion is, and has always been, to help people take a preventive approach to their health: a full lifestyle change that includes proper diet, regular exercise and less dependence on prescription medicines. I'm a bit of an exception, rather than the norm, with that lifestyle philosophy. When I designed the 17 Day Diet, I wanted to make sure it supported my prevention philosophy whilst giving people a programme that was sustainable. By all accounts that goal is being achieved. This cookbook is another tool you can use in your quest for a healthier weight and a healthier life.

I did not put it together on my own. I'd like to thank two superb cooks, Bruce Weinstein and Mark Scarborough, for their contributions. Bruce and Mark grasped the concepts of the diet immediately and were able to turn the 17 Day Diet foods into delicious, easy-to-make recipes that will become a part of your everyday life. Thanks are also due to Maggie Greenwood-Robinson for guiding the project, and to the entire amazing team at Free Press, including Leah Miller and Dominick Anfuso, for having the vision and creativity to bring this cookbook about.

CONTENTS

INTRODUCTION

Quick show of hands: how many people have rapidly lost a significant amount of weight on the 17 Day Diet? Let's see, that's one, two, three . . . uh, looks like lots of people.

Now, I'm happy to say that you're going to be able lose even more weight and enjoy it even more with this brand-new cookbook.

Introducing *The 17 Day Diet Cookbook*.

Before you start to panic, rest assured that you don't need to shout and jump and spin knives, make meals that look like a major work of art or get a degree from Le Cordon Bleu. All you need are some easy-to-follow, easy-to-prepare recipes that are extraordinarily delicious. This cookbook gives you all that and more.

Most of the recipes can be prepared in 30 minutes or less. There are no long lists of ingredients, complicated cooking methods, or hard-to-understand directions. All the recipes are built around the foods you eat on the 17 Day Diet.

The 17 Day Diet is a 4-cycle nutrition programme that makes it fast and easy to lose weight, without feeling deprived or hungry all the time. With this companion cookbook, you'll have delectable recipes at your fingertips so you can lose even more weight without giving up delicious foods. It's the perfect way for people with refined palates to lose weight and get healthy. As a family doctor and an advocate of preventive health, I believe healthy food can still be wonderful. I refuse to accept that a diet has to involve going to extremes or that diet food has to taste like cardboard. It doesn't! It just has to be thoughtfully prepared, in a reasonable amount of time, and taste incredibly good. That's the kind of food you'll find in this book.

I encourage you to try several of these recipes each week to reap the benefits. Broken record, I know, but if you're going to eat healthily and lose more weight, you need to cook more at home. When you do, you have control over what you eat and more control over how much weight you ultimately lose. My nutrition team has developed recipes that taste good and are high in nutrition. We use ingredients that are mainly found in your average supermarket. Use these recipes, and you may never feel like you're on a diet, either!

What I enjoyed most about putting this cookbook together was that I got to sample and test new recipes before they appeared in this book. Some of my favourites are Polynesian Grilled Beef, Tuscan Pork Tenderloin, Crab Cakes, Open-faced Reuben, Spiced Edamame Soya Beans, Microwave Mashed Potatoes, Mexican Chocolate Pudding, Chocolatey Frozen Yoghurt . . . well, I could go on and on. They're all my favourites!

I'd like to emphasize, too, that cooking at home can also save you a bundle, because you'll likely spend less buying groceries than eating out, and it can even make dating cheaper. After all, who isn't impressed by a partner who knows how to cook? Restaurants must charge high prices in order to pay their employees and other bills. If you cook at home, you design the menu and keep the tips yourself! For health and wealth, there's just no match for a good home-cooked meal, so please start serving more of them.

Home cooking isn't rocket science, either. Lots of us cook and eat. And lots of us love to talk about cooking and eating. With the increase in cookery programmes on TV, as a nation we're becoming more obsessed with food.

Personally, I just love food. Food and I go way back, more than 43 years now. One of my favourite ways to relax from a day at my surgery is to come home, roll up my sleeves and heat up the oven. I'm quite satisfied in the kitchen, experimenting with new recipes, sipping a glass of wine and enjoying what I've created. And you'll get to enjoy some of these creations right here in this book.

So, if you're in a dietary rut, want to lose even more weight or are in need of a little inspiration, *The 17 Day Diet Cookbook* is for you!

Refresher Course: The 17 Day Diet

The 17 Day Diet is a 4-cycle programme designed to take weight off rapidly. Isn't that what you want? Hardly anyone I know likes to endure depressingly slow weight loss. We want to be trim now, look great now and feel great now. The 17 Day Diet gets you to where you want to be quickly, without lots of sacrifice, hunger pangs or cravings. The diet is nutritionally sound, easy to follow and it works. I call it the best thing since the sliced bread you'll give up (but only for the first 2 cycles).

Trust me, this is a phenomenal diet. I've had people lose 4.5 to 5.5 kg (10 to 12 lb) over the first 17 days, and kept losing steadily right down to their goals. Of course, individuals do vary in their results. The beauty of this programme is that you won't get discouraged or bored by the prospect of staying on a diet for what seems like for ever because you're shedding fat so quickly. You'll love the fact that in 7, 10 or 17 days, you'll be slimmer. And if your results are like so many others, you'll feel a lot lighter and have an absurd amount of energy.

Overview of the 4 Cycles

The beauty of the 17 Day Diet is that it works in 4 cycles, depending on how much weight you'd like to lose.

Cycle 1 is the initial 17 day period during which you give up all bread, rice, potatoes, pasta, baked goods, fruit, sweets, cake, ice cream and alcohol. It's the strictest period, but also when the most rapid weight loss occurs. And it's easier than you think. You won't even miss carbs after a few days, because your body gets used to not relying on them. You get to eat unlimited amounts of certain proteins and vegetables. And you'll supplement your daily diet with probiotics like yoghurt and kefir, foods shown in research to help the body burn fat.

The great thing about Cycle 1 is that you can use it anytime: when you need to break a plateau, get back to your goal weight, fit into a smaller dress size for the weekend or a swimming costume for a cruise, anytime you want to accelerate your weight loss and do it safely. Cycle 1 is one of your best quick-weight loss resources.

During Cycle 2, you slowly begin to reintroduce certain carbs, such as pulses, wholegrains and starchy vegetables, along with lots of other foods. Weight loss continues, and still fairly rapidly. And now you can drink a little wine, something most diets forbid.

On Cycle 3 you get to eat a huge of array of healthy foods: breads, more meats, more starches and fun foods like low-carb frozen dessert treats. You ease off some of the strictness of the first 2 cycles, whilst still continuing to knock off pounds. Every 17 days you're changing things round, so you never get bored. Every day is exciting because you see the results on your scales or in your more loosely fitting clothes.

Cycle 4 is the maintenance period that, ideally, you stay on the rest of your life. It lets you stay at your new weight as long as you do two things: enjoy yourself on the weekend, and use your favourite cycle during the week. So, once you're happy with your new svelte self, continue to enjoy occasional forbidden foods. Just do so carefully or you'll find yourself back on a slippery slope to your pre-diet weight. If you fall off the wagon for a weekend or, say, on a holiday, don't panic. Just jump back to Cycle 1 to quickly shave off any weight you gain.

Why the 17 Day Diet Works So Well

Eliminating unhealthy foods from your system keeps them from making a beeline to your tummy and elsewhere. Healthy foods do the opposite. The higher amounts of lean protein you eat on this diet, for example, boost your metabolism in a number of physiologically active ways. This diet is high in fibre, too, which is an appetite suppressant, a detoxifier and a food component that ushers bad calories out of your system before they have time to camp out on your thighs. Then there is the addition of probiotics, now believed to keep fat formation in check.

Another reason that the 17 Day Diet works is because you're changing your calorie count and the foods you eat. By varying these things you keep your body and metabolism guessing. I call this *body confusion*. The scales are less likely to get stuck. The added bonus: you'll never get bored. And it's fun watching those pounds melt off. So, confusion is good!

But, more importantly, the 17 Day Diet works because it's realistic and sustainable. Nothing derails a diet faster than distressing round-the-clock hunger pangs, or boredom. But the 17 Day Diet isn't about depriving yourself of food or variety. I encourage you to eat until you are no longer hungry, even snack between meals, as long as you're eating the right foods. That doesn't mean just broccoli, either. Nuts, cheeses and other delicious foods are permitted as you progress through the cycles. There are so many choices, too, that you'll never get bored.

Let's Start Cooking and Losing

You've read this and you're a believer, and you can't wait to get started. To learn all the intricacies of how and why the diet works, you need to get the book, *The 17 Day Diet*, and its other companion book, *The 17 Day Diet Workbook*. If you can't get to the bookshop straight away, here's an overview of the diet:

Quick and Easy Overview of the 17 Day Diet	
Cycle	**Purpose**
Cycle 1: Accelerate (17 days)	To promote rapid weight loss by improving digestive health. This cycle helps clear sugar from the blood to boost fat-burning and discourage fat storage.
Cycle 2: Activate (17 days)	To reset your metabolism through a strategy that involves increasing and decreasing your caloric consumption to stimulate fat-burning, and to help prevent plateaus.

Cycle 3: Achieve (17 days)	To develop good eating habits through the reintroduction of additional foods and move you closer to your goal weight.
Cycle 4: Arrive (ongoing)	To keep you at your goal weight through a programme of eating that lets you enjoy your favourite foods on weekends, whilst eating healthfully during the week.

How to Use This Cookbook

For losing weight on *The 17 Day Diet* this cookbook is divided into three easy-to-digest sections:

- Cycle 1 Recipes and Cycle 1 17 Day Meal Plan

- Cycle 2 Recipes and Cycle 2 17 Day Meal Plan

- Cycle 3 Recipes and Cycle 3 17 Day Meal Plan

Each section features delicious breakfasts, lunches, dinners and snacks that match the cycle you're in. I show you how to use those recipes by giving you menu plans for each cycle. That's a total of 51 daily menus to help you.

Follow these delicious meal plans, week by week. They will give you structure, which helps guard against unplanned eating, plus you can learn about some new foods and ways to prepare them. The meal plans are low in fat, high in fibre, packed with nutrition and designed to trigger rapid weight loss. I strongly believe that the way you eat to control your weight must continue for the rest of your life. These meal plans can help you do that. They provide a lifelong foundation for a healthy, enjoyable and satisfying way of eating.

Now that you're acquainted with how the 17 Day Diet works in conjunction with this cookbook, it's time to take action. People who have used this plan have told us they could not believe how effortless it was to lose weight and keep it off. Why? Because the 17 Day Diet is a way of life. Unlike your past dieting experiences, you'll never need to quit. As long as you keep going, you'll see results. Beginning in Cycle 1 you'll start to shed unwanted pounds and renew your vitality.

I know you'll enjoy what we've cooked up here. These are recipes that can satisfy your appetite and help you drop pounds. Each one has been created to help you succeed at getting your weight under control without skimping on the flavours you love.

I know you want meals that are quick and healthy. You want them to taste wonderful, you want them to help you lose weight and you want them now! Seems like a tall order, but that's what these recipes deliver, especially if you're prepared. Just start with a cycle's worth of meals and do it. Having the right ingredients to hand, plus kitchen equipment that makes preparation easier, will make cooking quicker and more healthful.

Time-savers are built into each recipe, too. For example, they take advantage of healthy convenience foods available in supermarkets, such as boneless, skinless chicken breasts. All you have to do is apply the finishing touches. For side dishes you'll use quick-cooking staples such as washed salad leaves, frozen fruits and vegetables, and quality convenience products, such as preprepared salad dressings and low-calorie condiments.

Preparing the 17 Day Diet recipes requires no special equipment, although some appliances (suggested but not required) can help, and these are listed for you here. There are few meals that can't be made leaner or healthier by using cooking methods such as grilling, steaming, baking, lightly stir-frying, microwaving and sautéing in water or with vegetable cooking spray. With every new recipe you try, you will discover low-fat and low-carb cooking tips, healthy methods of food preparation, ways to cut the fat, sugar, calories and cholesterol, and how to use fresh herbs and spices to add flavour. We also include important information on kitchen tools that can help you prepare healthful meals. You may already have lots of the equipment in your kitchen. The rest you should be able to pick up at any kitchen shop or kitchen department in larger department stores. Consider these tools to help you get your weight under control. The more weight-loss tools you have, the more successful you will be.

Pots and Pans

Look for heavy pots and pans, preferably with nonstick coatings and tight-fitting lids. The nonstick coating can help you cut down the amount of oil or other fats you need to coat the pan, and it'll make washing up a lot easier.

Saucepans: at least three
(a 1-litre/1¾-pint pan, a 2-litre/3½-pint pan and a 3-litre/5¼-pint pan)

Frying pans: two or three
(a 20-cm/8-inch pan and a 30-cm/12-inch pan)

Soup pot: a 5- or 6-litre/8½- or 10-pint pot

Utensils

Stocking your kitchen with the following utensils will make your culinary efforts easier and more enjoyable. You may even find that having a couple of sets of some items, such as wooden spoons and palette knives, is more convenient than having to wash the tools several times throughout the preparation of a meal.

Colander

Chopping board

Egg separator

Garlic press

Grater

Kitchen scissors

Palette knives and fish slice

Sieve

Timer

Whisks

Wooden spoons

Other Useful Items

If you have the storage space in your kitchen, these additional items are less essential, but definitely helpful.

Baking tins: a 33- x 23- x 5-cm/13- x 9- x 2-inch tin;
a 20- x 20- x 5-cm/8- x 8- x 2-inch tin

Bun tin: one or two

Wine cooling rack: preferably a large, square one, for cooling bread and muffins. A rack permits the air to circulate, reducing sogginess.

Ovenproof dishes: at least two (a 1½-litre/2½-pint dish and a 3-litre/5-pint dish), with covers

Mixing bowls: several sizes

Slow cooker: good for soups and lean cuts of meats

Steamer: for cooking vegetables and reheating foods that do best with moist heat

Wok: for stir-frying and steaming

The 17 Day Diet
COOKBOOK

RECIPES

Cycle 1 – Accelerate

GOAL: To trigger rapid weight loss in a healthy manner by mobilising fat stores and flushing water and toxins from your system.

Snappy Eggs

Skipping breakfast is not a good idea. People who miss breakfast are more likely to overeat at other times throughout the day and gain weight. I realise that you might not have lots of time in the morning, but here's a recipe that will let you enjoy a great breakfast even if you're rushed for time.

INGREDIENTS
500 g/1 lb 2 oz preprepared salsa
4 medium eggs

DIRECTIONS
1. Position a rack in the middle of the oven and preheat to Gas Mark 6/200°C/fan oven 180°C. Spoon the salsa into a 20-cm/8-inch ovenproof dish. Set in the oven and heat for 15 minutes.

2. Remove the ovenproof dish from the oven. Use the back of a wooden spoon to create 4 evenly spaced wells in the salsa. Crack an egg into each of these wells. Return to the oven and bake until the whites are set but the yolks are still soft, for 8 to 10 minutes. (For hard-cooked yolks, bake for 15 minutes.) Use a large spoon to scoop the eggs into serving bowls along with the hot salsa.

YIELD: 2 servings (can be doubled using a 23- x 33-cm/9- x 13-inch ovenproof dish)

> **TIPS:** Heat the salsa whilst you take a shower! There are lots of salsas on the market so you can customise the eggs to your taste. Peach salsa. Extra hot salsa. Experiment!

Spanish Omelette

Being of Hispanic descent, I love fluffy Spanish omelettes. Add a couple of fresh jalapeño slices for more zip. The egg whites here cut the fat and calories and also make it a healthy, high-protein dish.

INGREDIENTS
1 egg
2 egg whites
⅛ teaspoon salt
⅛ teaspoon black pepper
1 tablespoon olive oil
60 g/2¼ oz tomato, chopped
15 g/½ oz diced onion
15 g/½ oz fat-free Cheddar cheese, grated

DIRECTIONS
1. In a medium bowl, whisk together egg, egg whites, salt and black pepper. Heat a frying pan over a medium-high heat.

2. Add olive oil and swirl the pan to coat the base and sides. Add eggs and tilt the pan to spread the mixture across the entire pan base. Cook for about 30 seconds.

3. With a palette knife, gently lift sides of omelette and tilt the pan to distribute more uncooked egg to the pan's surface. Once the egg begins to set, sprinkle diced tomato, onion and Cheddar cheese over one side of the omelette. Carefully fold the other side of the omelette over the fillings.

YIELD: 1 serving

Mushroom Spinach Frittata

To me eggs are everything they're cracked up to be. I absolutely love them in any way, shape or form. Here's one of my favourite egg recipes. I've had it for breakfast, lunch and dinner. If you've never had breakfast for dinner, you have no idea what you're missing!

INGREDIENTS

3 medium eggs

2 medium egg whites

280 g/10 oz chopped spinach, thawed if frozen

2 teaspoons olive oil

175 g/6 oz white or chestnut mushrooms, thinly sliced

1 tablespoon finally chopped fresh oregano leaves or 1 teaspoon dried oregano

½ teaspoon salt

½ teaspoon ground black pepper

½ teaspoon dried chilli flakes, optional

DIRECTIONS

1. Use a fork or a whisk to beat the eggs and egg whites in a small bowl until creamy and thick. Set aside.

2. Squeeze the chopped spinach by handfuls over the sink to remove excess moisture. Set aside.

3. Heat the olive oil in a 25-cm/10-inch, non-stick frying pan over a medium heat. Add the mushrooms and cook, stirring often, until they give off some of their liquid and it then evaporates, for about 5 minutes.

4. Crumble in the spinach and stir in the oregano, salt, pepper and chilli flakes. Stir for 2 minutes to warm the spinach and toast the spices.

5. Beat the eggs one more time to ensure they're creamy, then pour them into the frying pan. Reduce the heat to low, cover and cook

(continued on next page)

until set and no longer runny for about 10 minutes. Loosen the frittata with a heat-safe rubber palette knife and slide on to a chopping board to slice into quarters.

YIELD: 2 servings

TIP: Put the frozen chopped spinach in the fridge the night before to thaw.

Greek Egg Scramble

Enjoy this quick-to-make feast, with flavours that are a great way to start the day. I love Greek food so much, I should be Greek!

INGREDIENTS
Non-stick cooking spray
4 egg whites
100 g/3½ oz red onions, chopped
60 g/2¼ oz tomato, chopped
20 g/¾ oz reduced-fat feta cheese, crumbled
⅛ teaspoon salt
⅛ teaspoon black pepper

DIRECTIONS
1. In a medium bowl, combine all ingredients except non-stick spray.
2. Pour into a small frying pan that has been coated with non-stick spray.
3. Cook over a medium-low heat for 2 to 3 minutes, stirring frequently, until eggs are cooked through.

YIELD: 1 serving

Peach Melba Smoothie

Smoothies are a great way to sneak your fruit in, and give you plenty of nourishing vitamins, minerals and phytochemicals *(plant chemicals that contain protective, disease-preventing compounds). Whenever I crave something sweet, I go for a smoothie because it's perfectly satisfying and I feel totally energized afterwards. This recipe is a spectacular combination: hardly anything so nutritious tastes this good.*

INGREDIENTS

475 ml/16 fl oz plain, low-fat, unsweetened kefir

1 medium peach, peeled, stoned and sliced into wedges

125 g/4½ oz raspberries

1 teaspoon Truvia

⅛ teaspoon ground cinnamon

2 ice cubes

DIRECTIONS

Place all the ingredients in a blender, cover and blend until smooth. Divide into two glasses.

YIELD: 2 servings

TIPS: Use 175 g/6 oz frozen peach slices. You can save half the smoothie in a covered container in the fridge, for a snack later. Give it a whirl to make sure it's smooth before serving.

Kefir Smoothie

I like kefir. I've always liked the idea of fermented milk, which is healthy, natural and beneficial, but had never actually tried the stuff. I always thought it might be too sour for my tastes, so when I went shopping, I'd always look at it and think, "The kefir looks great", and then grab a litre of chocolate milk. I incorporated kefir into the 17 Day Diet because it's a fat-burning probiotic; now I love it, especially in smoothies.

INGREDIENTS

240 ml/8 fl oz unsweetened kefir
125 g/4½ oz frozen unsweetened berries
1 tablespoon sugar-free fruit jam or 1 tablespoon agave nectar
1 tablespoon linseed oil

DIRECTIONS

Place all ingredients in a blender and blend until smooth.

YIELD: 1 large serving

Yogurt Fruitshake

Don't worry: Acidophilus milk *might sound unappetising but it tastes just like ordinary milk. Plus, it gives you a healthy dose of probiotics to help you manage your weight.*

INGREDIENTS
125 ml/4 fl oz acidophilus milk
85 g/3 oz sugar-free fruit-flavoured yoghurt
125 g/4½ oz frozen unsweetened berries

DIRECTIONS
Place all ingredients in a blender and blend until smooth.

YIELD: 1 large serving

Chicken-Vegetable Soup

This is a water-based soup that offers lots of weight-control benefits such as helping to control hunger, reducing total calorie intake when eaten before or with a meal and filling you up. It's also a good source of nutrients you might fall short of.

INGREDIENTS

- 100 g/3½ oz cabbage, chopped
- 1 large carrot, chopped
- 225 g/8 oz okra, sliced
- 1 large onion, chopped
- 2 large celery sticks with leaves, chopped
- 400 g/14 oz canned chopped tomatoes
- 400 ml/14 fl oz fat-free chicken stock
- 1½ teaspoons salt
- ¼ teaspoon pepper
- 4 baked boneless, skinless chicken breasts, diced

DIRECTIONS

1. Place all ingredients except the chicken in a large pan and simmer for 1 hour, or until vegetables are soft.

2. Add the chicken and heat thoroughly.

YIELD: 4 servings

California Tuna Salad

Whether it's piled on top of a salad, stuffed in fresh tomatoes or slathered between two slices of wholemeal bread, I love tuna salad. However, it's important to prepare it so that you can control the amount of fat that goes into it. Translation: no creamy mayonnaise smothering the tuna! This version of tuna salad is low in fat, and oh so delicious, as well as easy to make. Please note: tuna tends to be high in mercury. My advice is to eat tuna no more than twice a week to be on the cautious side.

INGREDIENTS

2 tablespoons lemon juice

Up to 1½ tablespoons olive oil, optional

2 teaspoons Dijon mustard

½ teaspoon salt

½ teaspoon black pepper

185 g/6½ oz tuna canned in water, drained

235 g/8½ oz ready-prepared artichoke hearts bottled in water, drained, and halved

2 celery sticks, finely chopped

2 medium spring onions, thinly sliced

DIRECTIONS

Whisk the lemon juice, olive oil, if using, mustard, salt and pepper in a large bowl until smooth and creamy. Add the remaining ingredients and stir until combined and coated.

YIELD: 2 servings (can be doubled or tripled)

> **TIPS:** Serve on a bed of lettuce. For less fat, omit the lemon juice, olive oil, mustard, salt and pepper; use 60 ml/2 fl oz fat-free, no-carb honey, Dijon or creamy Italian dressing. If you love tuna salad, always keep a couple of cans in the refrigerator, so that when you make this salad, it's already cool.

Super Salad

Any diet that leaves you feeling hungry is doomed to fail. The 17 Day Diet will not do that. It's high in foods that make you feel full, like veggies. So have your fill of this salad, and it will keep you feeling full.

INGREDIENTS

Lettuce, any variety, torn into bite-sized pieces

Cucumbers

Onions

Tomatoes

Other salad vegetables such as celery, peppers or raw broccoli

2 hard-boiled eggs, peeled and chopped

2 tablespoons olive or linseed oil

60 ml/2 fl oz balsamic vinegar

DIRECTIONS

1. Combine lettuce with vegetables and hard-boiled eggs.

2. Toss with olive or linseed oil and balsamic vinegar.

3. Season to taste.

YIELD: 1 serving

Turkey Picadillo Lettuce Wraps

Want a suitable substitute for bread? Try lettuce wraps. They make great sandwiches, they're more filling than bread (because lettuce is high in water volume) and keep your carb intake down to practically zero.

INGREDIENTS

Non-stick cooking spray

1 medium white onion, chopped

1 medium garlic clove, finely chopped

1 medium red pepper, deseeded and chopped

450 g/1 lb lean turkey mince

1 large tomato, roughly chopped

15 g/½ oz fresh parsley leaves, finely chopped, or 2 tablespoons dried parsley flakes

1 tablespoon finely chopped fresh oregano leaves or 1 teaspoon dried oregano

1 tablespoon chilli powder

1 tablespoon Worcestershire sauce

½ teaspoon cinnamon

1½ teaspoons apple-cider vinegar

8 Cos or Little Gem lettuce leaves, thick stems removed

DIRECTIONS

1. Spray a large frying pan with non-stick cooking spray. Set over a medium heat for 1 minute. Add onion and garlic. Cook, stirring occasionally, until softened, for about 3 minutes. Add the red pepper; continue cooking, stirring occasionally, for about 2 minutes

2. Add the turkey mince, and break up with a spoon. Cook, stirring frequently, until lightly browned, for about 6 minutes.

3. Raise the heat to medium-high. Stir in the tomato, parsley, oregano, chilli powder, Worcestershire sauce and cinnamon. Cook, stirring occasionally, until the tomatoes break down, their liquid evaporates and the frying pan is almost dry, for about 5 minutes. Remove from the heat and stir in the vinegar. Cool for 10 minutes,

then spoon filling equally into each lettuce leaf, roll the leaves up and serve.

YIELD: 4 servings

TIPS: For a packed lunch, pack the picadillo and the lettuce leaves separately. To save prep time look in the produce section of your supermarket for prepared peppers and even onions.

Lemon-Pepper Salmon Salad in Tomato Cups

This super-low-fat salmon salad with fresh tomatoes looks and is delicious enough to serve when you're entertaining. Don't assume that means being tied up for hours in the kitchen. You can make this salad fast and ahead of time. And if there's one food I could live on, it's salmon. It's full of omega-3 fatty acids, which are good for brain function and for combating inflammation and stiffness.

INGREDIENTS

175 g/6 oz canned salmon, drained

2 celery sticks, finely chopped

60 g/2¼ oz fat-free soured cream

15 g/½ oz white onion, finely chopped

1 teaspoon lemon-pepper seasoning

2 large tomatoes

DIRECTIONS

1. Mix the salmon, celery, soured cream, onion and lemon-pepper seasoning in a small bowl.

2. Slice 5 mm/¼ inch off the stalk end of each tomato. Use a melon baller to scoop out the seeds and membranes, leaving 2 tomato cups. Spoon half the salmon salad into each cup to serve.

YIELD: 2 servings (can be doubled or tripled)

> **TIPS:** For the best taste, look for wild-caught, skinless, boneless pink salmon. To finely chop celery, cut the sticks lengthways into thin strips, then slice these as thinly as possible. For a packed lunch, pack the salad and tomatoes separately. The salad can stay covered in the fridge for up to 3 days, but not in the tomato cups.

Creamy Smoked Salmon Rolls

Bagels are a traditional accompaniment to smoked salmon and cream cheese, but since you can't eat bagels until later on the diet, here's an amazing alternative that will satisfy your taste buds whilst waiting.

INGREDIENTS
- 115 g/4 oz thinly sliced smoked salmon
- 115 g/4 oz yoghurt cheese made from fat-free, natural Greek yoghurt (see recipe overleaf)
- ½ teaspoon fresh dill
- ½ teaspoon finely grated lemon zest
- ¼ teaspoon garlic powder
- 1 large cucumber, sliced into 5-mm/¼-inch circles

DIRECTIONS
1. Lay a large piece of greaseproof paper on your work surface. Lay the smoked salmon slices on the greaseproof paper, overlapping them to make a large rectangle. Spread the yogurt cheese on top of the salmon, then sprinkle evenly with the dill, lemon zest and garlic powder. Using the greaseproof paper to lift the salmon up, roll the fish like a Swiss roll, taking care that the greaseproof paper is only a guide and doesn't get caught inside the roll. Wrap the log in cling film, then refrigerate for at least 1 hour or up to 24 hours.

2. Unwrap the roll and lay on a chopping board. Use a serrated knife to slice into 1-cm/½-inch-thick pinwheels. Place each piece on top of a cucumber circle.

YIELD: 2 servings

TIP: Make ahead, slice off as much of the log as you want, then rewrap the rest of the log and refrigerate.

Yoghurt Cheese

This easy-to-make cheese can be enjoyed as a tangy dip for vegetables or, in later cycles, as a topping for jacket potatoes. It is completely fat free and tastes just like high-fat soured cream.

INGREDIENTS
900 g/2 lb fat-free Greek yoghurt
Spices, such as coarse salt, garlic or oregano

DIRECTIONS
1. Line a sieve with a coffee filter or white kitchen paper. Place the sieve over a bowl to catch the liquid. Spoon in the fat-free yoghurt.

2. Cover and refrigerate for 8 hours or overnight.

3. Makes about 450 g/1 lb of yoghurt cheese. Mix in your favourite spices for a tangy dip for vegetables or use as a topping for jacket potatoes.

Stir-fried Chicken and Cucumbers

The best fast food around is stir-fry. Granted, there may be some chopping involved, but that's a small price to pay for a delicious hot meal you can serve this quickly.

INGREDIENTS

Non-stick cooking spray

6 medium spring onions, thinly sliced

1 tablespoon peeled fresh ginger, finely chopped

1 medium garlic clove, finely chopped

450 g/1 lb boneless skinless chicken breasts, thinly sliced

2 medium cucumbers, halved lengthways, deseeded and thinly sliced

2 tablespoons light soy sauce

2 tablespoons unseasoned rice vinegar

Up to 1 teaspoon Tabasco sauce, optional

DIRECTIONS

1. Spray a large wok or frying pan with non-stick cooking spray and set over a medium-high heat until smoking. Add the spring onions, ginger and garlic. Toss and stir over the heat for 30 seconds.

2. Add the chicken strips. Toss and stir until lightly browned and any trace of pink is gone, for about 3 minutes.

3. Add the cucumbers. Stir-fry until heated through and softening at the edges, for about 2 minutes. Pour in the soy sauce, rice vinegar and Tabasco sauce, if using. Stir until bubbling, until the chicken has absorbed some of the sauce, for less than 1 minute.

YIELD: 4 servings

(continued on next page)

Stir-fried Chicken and Cucumbers (*cont.*)

TIPS: For an even quicker meal, look in the chiller cabinet for sliced boneless skinless chicken breast fillets, sometimes sold as chicken for stir-fries.

No need to peel cucumbers if they are organic or from a farmer's market. However, cucumbers from the supermarket may have been waxed with a food-grade wax and should be peeled for the best-tasting dish. Unwaxed cucumbers are sold in a shrink-wrapped plastic film.

Rice vinegar needs a note. Unseasoned rice vinegar is just rice vinegar, usually not labelled as anything other than rice vinegar. 'Seasoned' rice vinegar includes sugar. Make sure you have unseasoned; look at the ingredient list on the bottle's label.

You can use Tabasco or a similar hot sauce. I really like the Indonesian sambal olek, which is banging hot. It's now available in the Asian section of almost every supermarket.

Tandoori Chicken Breasts

I love Indian food, and this traditional tandoori chicken fits the bill. The chicken is marinated in yoghurt and spices, then cooked to perfection. Yoghurt, a key fat-burning ingredient in the 17 Day Diet, is very popular in Indian and Middle Eastern cooking, both in sauces and side dishes to help soothe the tongue whilst eating spicy dishes.

INGREDIENTS

75 g/2½ oz natural, low-fat yoghurt or natural, low-fat kefir
1 tablespoon curry powder
½ teaspoon Truvia
¼ teaspoon garlic powder
4 boneless skinless chicken breasts, about 115 g/4 oz each
Non-stick cooking spray
625 g/1½ lbs baby spinach leaves, washed but not dried

DIRECTIONS

1. Mix the yoghurt, curry powder, Truvia and garlic powder in a large bowl to make a wet paste. Add the chicken breasts, stir and toss until well coated. Cover and store in the fridge for at least 30 minutes or up to 4 hours.

2. Spray a griddle pan with non-stick cooking spray and set over a medium-high heat. Alternatively, spray a large baking tray with non-stick cooking spray, set it on the oven shelf 10 to 15 cm/4 to 6 inches from the grill and preheat the grill.

3. Place the chicken breasts on the grilled pan or the baking tray. (Do not wipe off the marinade.) Grill for 8 minutes, turning once, until browned and cooked through. Transfer the cooked chicken to a chopping board.

4. Dump the wet spinach into a large saucepan and set over a medium heat. Cook, tossing often, until the spinach begins to wilt and steam from the moisture, about 2 minutes. Divide the spinach

(continued on next page)

Tandoori Chicken Breasts (*cont.*)

between four serving plates. Slice the chicken into strips and fan these out over the spinach.

YIELD: 4 servings

> **TIPS:** This dish can also be served with Oven-roasted Cauliflower and Broccoli (page 34). Greek yoghurt is too thick for this dish. Use ordinary yoghurt or kefir to coat the chicken breasts. There is an astounding array of curry powders on the market. Search for big-flavoured varieties in the international aisle of most large supermarkets, or look for one to your taste at Indian supermarkets or online.

Low-carb Primavera Delight

Who needs noodles when you've got spaghetti squash? This low-carb dish will fill you up without filling you out, and you won't even miss the pasta.

INGREDIENTS

1 spaghetti squash or butternut squash
185 g/6½ oz broccoli, chopped
1 small onion, diced
2 garlic cloves, finely chopped
1 tablespoon olive oil
Tomato pasta sauce, for serving, heated

DIRECTIONS

1. Preheat the oven to Gas Mark 5/190°C/fan oven 170°C. To prepare the squash, cut it in half. Scoop out the seeds and pulp as you would any squash or pumpkin.

2. Place squash, rind side up, in a glass ovenproof dish filled with about 1 cm/½ inch of water. Bake for 40 to 45 minutes, or microwave the squash for 8 to 10 minutes per half on high.

3. Let the squash stand for a few minutes after cooking. Separate strands by running a fork through it lengthwise. Place strands in a bowl. Alternatively, if using the butternut squash, scoop out bite-sized pieces.

4. Whilst the squash is cooking, in a medium frying pan set over a medium-high heat, cook the broccoli, onion, garlic and oil until the vegetables are crisp-tender, stirring constantly, for about 4 minutes. Add the squash and heat thoroughly. Serve on plates topped with the pasta sauce.

YIELD: 4 servings

No-fuss Aubergine Parmesan

Aubergine Parmesan, an Italian standby, is one of my favourite dishes. We developed this quick version so that I could have it more often. It's super low in carbs and fat, and you won't even miss the breading.

INGREDIENTS

Non-stick cooking spray

1 large aubergine, trimmed and sliced into 1-cm/½-inch-thick rounds

450 g/1 lb lean turkey mince

1 kg/2 lb 4 oz low-carb ready-prepared tomato pasta sauce

1½ tablespoons finely chopped fresh oregano leaves or 2 teaspoons dried oregano

1 teaspoon fennel seeds

125 g/4½ oz fat-free cheese, such as Parmesan, freshly grated

DIRECTIONS

1. Position a rack in the centre of the oven and preheat to Gas Mark 4/180°C/fan oven 160°C. Spray a large baking tray with non-stick cooking spray. Lay the aubergine slices on the baking tray and spray them lightly with non-stick cooking spray. Bake, turning once, until the slices begin to soften and brown, for about 30 minutes.

2. Meanwhile, spray a large saucepan with non-stick cooking spray. Set over a medium heat and add the turkey mince, breaking it up with a spoon. Cook, stirring often, until the meat loses its raw, pink colour and browns a bit, for about 5 minutes. Pour in the tomato pasta sauce, then stir in the oregano and fennel seeds. Remove the pan from the heat.

3. Layer the aubergine slices and turkey pasta sauce in a 23- x 33-cm/9- x 13-inch ovenproof dish. Sprinkle the cheese on top. Bake until bubbling, for about 30 minutes. Cool for 5 minutes before serving.

YIELD: 4 servings

Curried Poached Halibut

Whilst grilling, *or holding a chunk of meat above a fire, might be the oldest form of cookery,* poaching, *or cooking in simmering liquid was probably not far behind. For a simple dinner, a poached fillet of fish served with a sauce made by reducing the cooking liquid is fast and easy.*

INGREDIENTS
350 ml/12 fl oz fat-free, reduced-sodium chicken stock

1 large leek, white and pale green parts only, halved lengthways, rinsed thoroughly, and thinly sliced

1 large red pepper, deseeded, and chopped

270 g/9½ oz small cauliflower florets

1 tablespoon peeled, finely chopped, fresh root ginger or ready-prepared finely chopped root ginger

1 tablespoon curry powder

4 skinless halibut fillets, about 115 g/4 oz each

115 g/4 oz low-fat natural yoghurt

1 teaspoon lemon juice

DIRECTIONS

1. Pour the stock into a large, deep frying pan or a wide, deep saucepan. Stir in the leeks, red pepper, cauliflower, ginger and curry powder. Set over a medium heat and bring to a low simmer. Cover, reduce heat to low and simmer for 5 minutes.

2. Place the fillets into the stock mixture. Cover and continue simmering until the fish is cooked through and flakes when tested with a fork, for 8 to 10 minutes.

3. Use a slotted spoon or a fish slice to transfer the fish to four serving bowls. Remove the pan from the heat and stir the yoghurt and lemon juice into the sauce. Divide the sauce between the bowls.

(continued on next page)

Curried Poached Halibut (*cont.*)

> **TIPS:** Slice larger cauliflower florets into smaller even-sized pieces so they cook faster. Look for ready-prepared ginger in tubes in the produce section. Refrigerate for freshness after opening. You can also buy frozen chopped ginger in handy cubes.

Griddled Tuna Niçoise Salad

The Niçoise salad is a French classic from Nice. It's usually made with hard-boiled eggs, anchovies, black olives, tomatoes and so forth. Our version uses lots of Cycle 1 veggies instead, to cut the calories but not the flavour.

INGREDIENTS

- 450 g/1 lb tuna steak, about 1 cm/½ inch thick
- 2 teaspoons olive oil
- ½ teaspoon salt
- ½ teaspoon black pepper
- 450 g/1 lb small cauliflower florets
- 350 g/12 oz green beans, topped and tailed and cut into 2.5-cm/1-inch pieces
- 350 g/12 oz small asparagus spears, cut into 2.5-cm/1-inch pieces
- 12 cherry tomatoes, halved
- 125 ml/4 fl oz fat-free, low-carb, ready-prepared French dressing
- 1 medium head Cos lettuce, cored, and leaves torn into small pieces

DIRECTIONS

1. Rub the tuna steak with the olive oil on both sides and sprinkle with salt and pepper. Heat a large griddle pan over a medium-high heat. Add the tuna and cook until medium-rare for about 6 minutes, turning once. (Cook for about 8 minutes for well-done.) Transfer to a chopping board.

2. Bring a large saucepan of water to a boil over a high heat. Add the cauliflower, green beans and asparagus. Cook for 3 minutes. Drain in a colander. Rinse with cool water to stop the cooking process, then drain well. Transfer the vegetables to a large bowl.

3. Cut the tuna into pieces about the size of the vegetables and add to the bowl. Add the tomatoes. Add the dressing and toss gently. Divide the Cos lettuce between four plates, then spoon a quarter of the griddled tuna salad on top of the lettuce on each plate.

YIELD: 4 servings

(continued on next page)

Griddled Tuna Niçoise Salad (*cont.*)

TIP: Try using ready-prepared low-carb, fat-free, sugar-free vinaigrette.

Oven-barbecued Chicken

I don't want to incur the wrath of barbecue purists by introducing this quick-to-make oven version, but I defy you to come away from the table without a glow of satisfied contentment after eating this. The chicken is just a bit sweet, thanks to the wonderful natural sweetener agave nectar, with a bit of heat that emphasizes the chicken flavour.

INGREDIENTS

Non-stick cooking spray

4 skinless boneless chicken breasts

200 g/7 oz reduced-sugar tomato ketchup

2 tablespoons Worcestershire sauce

1 tablespoon agave nectar

1 teaspoon chilli powder

DIRECTIONS

1. Preheat oven to Gas Mark 4/180°C/fan oven 160°C.

2. Place chicken breasts in a baking tin that has been sprayed with non-stick cooking spray.

3. Bake for 20 to 25 minutes.

4. In the meantime, stir together ketchup, Worcestershire sauce, agave nectar and chilli powder.

5. Remove chicken breasts from the oven and coat with the sauce. Return to the oven and bake for 10 minutes.

YIELD: 4 servings

Bavarian Chicken Breasts

You may have tried sauerkraut on a traditional, fattening and American-style Reuben sandwich, but try it like this too. Sauerkraut gets its name from two German words: sauer *(sour) and* kraut *(cabbage). Historically, it was part of sailors' diets to help prevent attacks of scurvy, because of the cabbage's vitamin C content. And by the way, I have a recipe for a Reuben sandwich on page 125 . . . it's delish and won't pack on pounds!*

INGREDIENTS

450 g/1 lb sauerkraut, rinsed and drained

12 medium Brussels sprouts, trimmed and cut in half lengthways

1 large tart green apple, peeled and coarsely grated

175 ml/6 fl oz fat-free, reduced-sodium chicken stock

1 teaspoon Dijon mustard

1 teaspoon caraway seeds

1 teaspoon dried dill

4 boneless skinless chicken breasts, about 115 g/4 oz each

2 teaspoons mild paprika

DIRECTIONS

1. Combine the sauerkraut, Brussels sprouts, apple, stock, mustard, caraway seeds and dill in a large, deep frying pan or saucepan. Bring to a boil over a medium heat, stirring occasionally. Cover, reduce the heat to low and simmer for 10 minutes.

2. Stir the sauerkraut mixture, then nestle the chicken breasts into it. Sprinkle the paprika over the chicken. Cover and continue simmering until the chicken is cooked through and the Brussels sprouts are tender, for about 20 minutes.

YIELD: 4 servings

> **TIP:** Look for jars of sauerkraut in the vegetable aisle in your supermarket.

Baked Tilapia Parcels

Looking to add something new to your seafood repertoire? Give tilapia a try. With recent attention focusing on the high contaminant levels of some fish, farm tilapia is a toxin-free and environmentally friendly alternative available in some supermarkets. Tilapia is a freshwater white fish with edible skin and a mild taste. It's very low in fat: a 175-g/6-oz serving contains less than 3 grams. And, because it is digested quickly, it is a great whole-food protein source to eat before or after workouts.

INGREDIENTS
    4 sheets kitchen foil, about 40 cm/16 inches each
    4 sheets baking parchment, about 40 cm/16 inches each
    4 skinless tilapia fillets, about 115 g/4 oz each
    2 medium red peppers, deseeded and chopped
    450 g/1 lb broccoli florets
    2 tablespoons chives, finely chopped
    2 tablespoons basil leaves, finely chopped
    1 large lemon, quartered
    ½ teaspoon salt

DIRECTIONS
1. Position a shelf in the centre of the oven and preheat to Gas Mark 8/230°C/fan oven 210°C.

2. Lay the sheets of foil on your work surface, then lay the sheets of baking parchment on top of the foil. Lay a tilapia fillet in the middle of each piece of baking parchment. Divide the red peppers, broccoli florets and herbs evenly between the servings. Squeeze lemon juice over each and sprinkle with salt. Seal the parcels, crimping the seams on each side. Set them on a large baking tray.

3. Bake for 15 minutes. Remove the baking tray from the oven and let stand at room temperature for 5 minutes. To serve, transfer each parcel to a plate and let each diner open their own – or open the parcels and transfer the contents to individual bowls.

YIELD: 4 servings

(continued on next page)

TIPS: Baking parchment is found next to kitchen foil in the supermarket. We don't recommend cooking acidic foods directly on kitchen foil. The parcels are hot. Make sure you open carefully so that the escaping steam doesn't burn you.

Any thin, white-fleshed fish fillet will work: red snapper, sea bass and so on. However, the fillets must be skinned. With the skin on the fish can curl up as it cooks.

DINNER

Blackened Mahi-Mahi

My love affair with Cajun cooking is too hot to cool down. You'll love this blackened fish, based on a recipe for catfish. Mahi-mahi is available at some upmarket supermarkets and from fishmongers. This is a healthy way to prepare the fish. Red pepper, asparagus and sugar snap peas add vitamins and phytonutrients. The flavour and tender, firm texture of this fish is an excellent and mahi-mahi is a good source of healthy, natural protein.

INGREDIENTS

- 4 skinless mahi-mahi or other firm white fish fillets, about 115 g/4 oz each
- 3 teaspoons sugar-free Cajun spice blend or seasoning mix
- 550 g/1 lb 4 oz cabbage, halved, cored and coarsely grated
- 1 large carrot, coarsely grated
- 125 ml/4 fl oz fat-free soured cream
- 1 tablespoon apple-cider vinegar

DIRECTIONS

1. Position the grill rack 10 to 15 cm/4 to 6 inches from the grill and preheat.

2. Rub each fish fillet with 1 teaspoon Cajun spice blend. Set on a baking tray or on the grill pan and grill for 8 minutes, turning once, until deeply browned and cooked through.

3. Meanwhile, combine the cabbage, carrot, soured cream, vinegar and the remaining 2 teaspoons of Cajun spice blend in a large bowl.

4. Divide the mixture evenly among 4 plates and transfer 1 fish fillet onto each pile of coleslaw.

> **TIP:** To save time, use 500 g/1 lb 2 oz of ready-prepared shredded cabbage instead of the cabbage. Use 125 ml/4 fl oz of calorie-free dressing instead of the soured cream and vinegar. Add the remaining Cajun spice blend to the bottled dressing to spice it up.

Oven-roasted Cauliflower and Broccoli

Fill up on fruits and veggies! Cruciferous vegetables such as broccoli, cauliflower and cabbage provide some defence against cancer. Broccoli was one of the first vegetables hailed for its anti-cancer properties, and it's still considered amongst the most potent. All three of these powerhouses contain sulphoraphane, a substance that defuses potential carcinogens.

INGREDIENTS
900 g/2 lb broccoli florets
680 g/1 lb 8 oz cauliflower florets
4 medium garlic cloves, quartered
1 tablespoon olive oil
½ teaspoon dried chilli flakes
½ teaspoon salt
1 tablespoon balsamic vinegar

DIRECTIONS
Position a shelf in the centre of the oven and preheat to Gas Mark 6/200°C/fan oven 180°C. Mix the broccoli, cauliflower, garlic, olive oil, chilli flakes, and salt in a large roasting tin or the grill pan. Roast, stirring and tossing occasionally, until the vegetables are crisp-tender and a little browned, for about 20 minutes. Remove from the oven, sprinkle with vinegar whilst still in the hot tin and toss well.

YIELD: 4 servings

Spicy Green Beans

Green beans are always good on their own . . . but spike them with garlic, chilli flakes, and ginger dressing, and they're great! This dish goes well with just about any main dish.

INGREDIENTS
2 teaspoons olive oil

3 medium garlic cloves, finely chopped

½ teaspoon dried chilli flakes

450 g/1 lb green beans, topped and tailed

2 tablespoons low-fat, low-carb, sugar-free sesame-ginger dressing

DIRECTIONS
1. Heat the oil in a frying pan or a wok over a medium-high heat. Add the garlic and chilli flakes and cook for 1 minute.

2. Add the green beans, then toss and stir over the heat until the beans are a little wilted, with dark brown spots, for about 4 minutes. Pour in the dressing and stir for 10 seconds until the green beans are coated and glazed.

YIELD: 4 servings

> **TIP:** Run the extractor fan over your hob or open a window. The volatile oils in the chilli flakes can be intense. Use standard green beans or dwarf green beans, not fine beans.

Balsamic Artichokes

One of the world's oldest medicinal plants, the artichoke is loaded with powerful antioxidants that promote health and assist in liver repair. I love pulling off those succulent leaves, dipping them in low-fat salad dressing and scraping the flesh from the leaf with my teeth. The closer you get to the 'heart' of the artichoke, the more tender the leaves are. Pull off the prickly pinkish parts and scrape the silk off the heart. The heart is the most delicious part; it takes work to get there, but it's definitely worth the effort.

INGREDIENTS
> 4 fresh artichokes
> 60 ml/2 fl oz balsamic vinegar
> Fat-free salad dressing

DIRECTIONS
1. In a large saucepan, bring 3–4 litres/5–7 pints of water to a boil and add balsamic vinegar. Add the artichokes, cover and cook for approximately 1 hour over a medium heat or until artichokes are tender, including the stem.

2. Let cool. Serve with fat-free salad dressing.

YIELD: 4 servings.

Green Tea-spiked Apple Sauce

Did you know that apples help prevent weight gain and even aid weight loss? It's true. They contain pectin, *a substance that delays stomach emptying, keeping you full longer. Pectin also lowers cholesterol almost as effectively as medicines do.*

INGREDIENTS

4 medium tart green apples, preferably Granny Smiths, peeled, cored and chopped

150 ml/5 fl oz strong, brewed green tea

2 teaspoons Truvia

10-cm/4-inch cinnamon stick

DIRECTIONS

Combine all the ingredients in a medium saucepan and bring to a bubble over a medium heat. Cover, reduce the heat to low and cook, stirring occasionally, until the apples are very tender for about 30 minutes. Discard the cinnamon stick. Mash into a thick purée with the back of a wooden spoon.

YIELD: 4 servings

TIP: The apple sauce can be served warm or cold. Leftovers can be stored in a covered container for up to 3 days. Even better, store in one-serving ramekins or containers.

Berry Frozen Yoghurt

Yes, you get to eat ice cream on the 17 Day Diet, and home-made, too. This frozen yoghurt is every bit as delectable as even high-quality ice cream.

INGREDIENTS

400 g/14 oz mixed berries, preferably about 140g/5 oz black-berries, 125 g/4½ oz raspberries and 140 g/5 oz blueberries

225 g/8 oz low-fat natural Greek yoghurt

1½ tablespoons Truvia

1 teaspoon lemon juice

⅛ teaspoon salt

DIRECTIONS

1. Place all the ingredients in a blender or food processor. Cover and process until smooth, turning off the machine and scraping down the inside of the container once or twice. Refrigerate for at least 1 hour or up to 1 day.

2. Freeze in an ice-cream machine according to the manufacturer's instructions.

YIELD: 4 servings

TIP: Use frozen mixed berries. Thaw and use them with their juices.

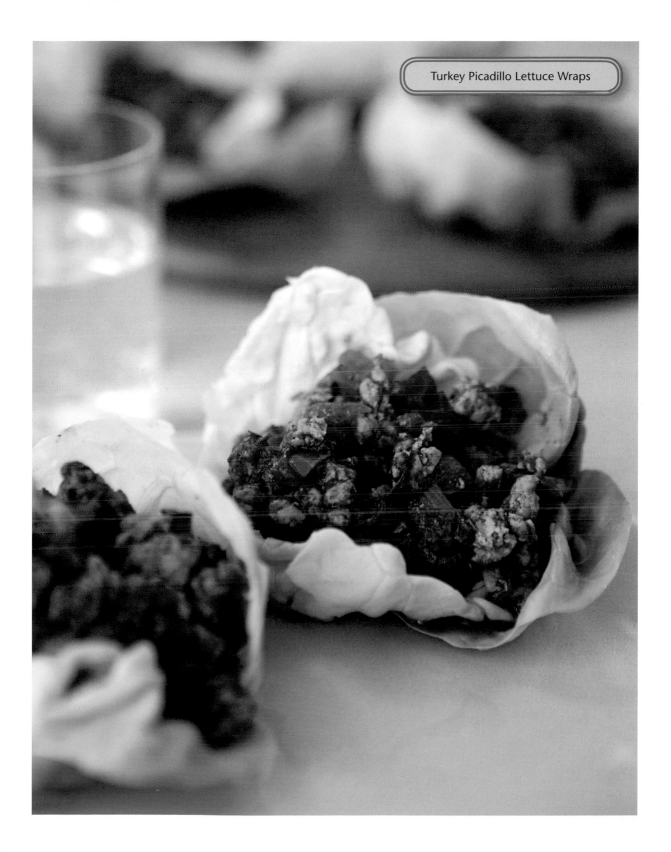

Turkey Picadillo Lettuce Wraps

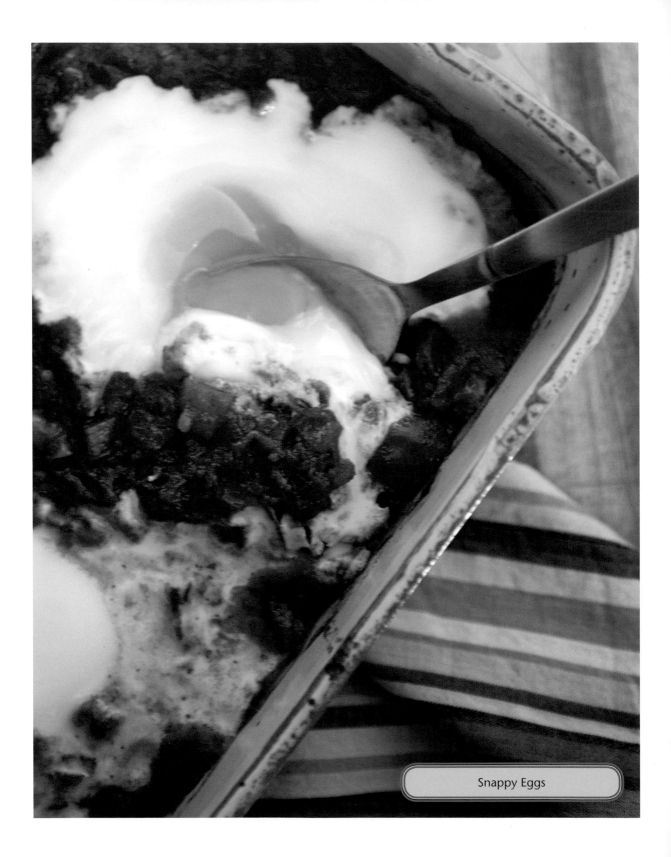

Snappy Eggs

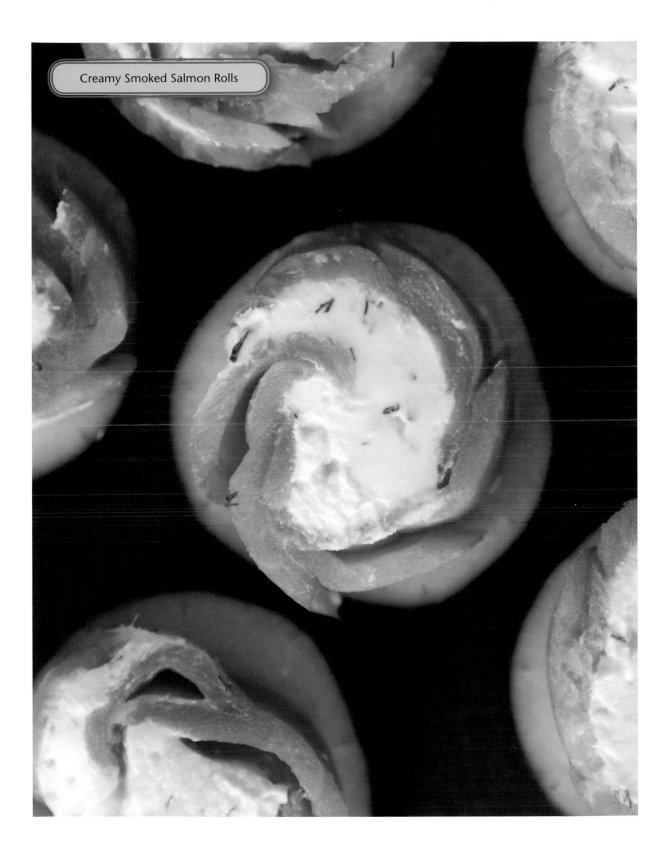

Creamy Smoked Salmon Rolls

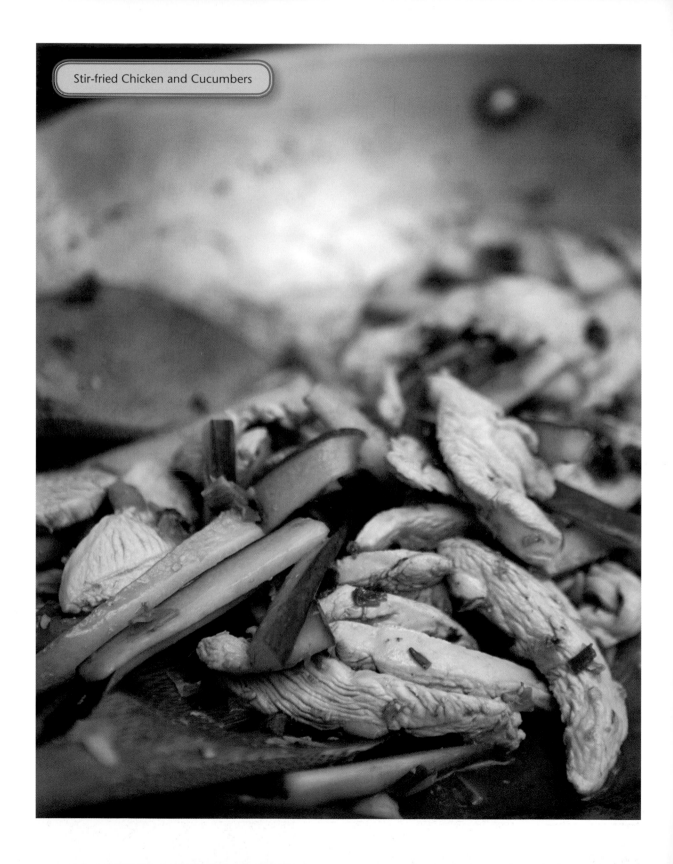

Stir-fried Chicken and Cucumbers

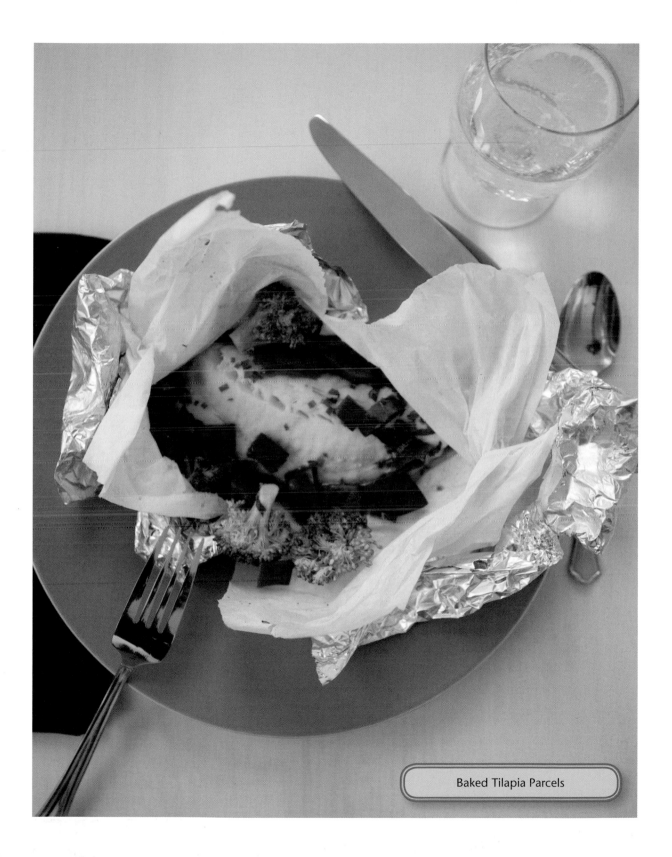

Baked Tilapia Parcels

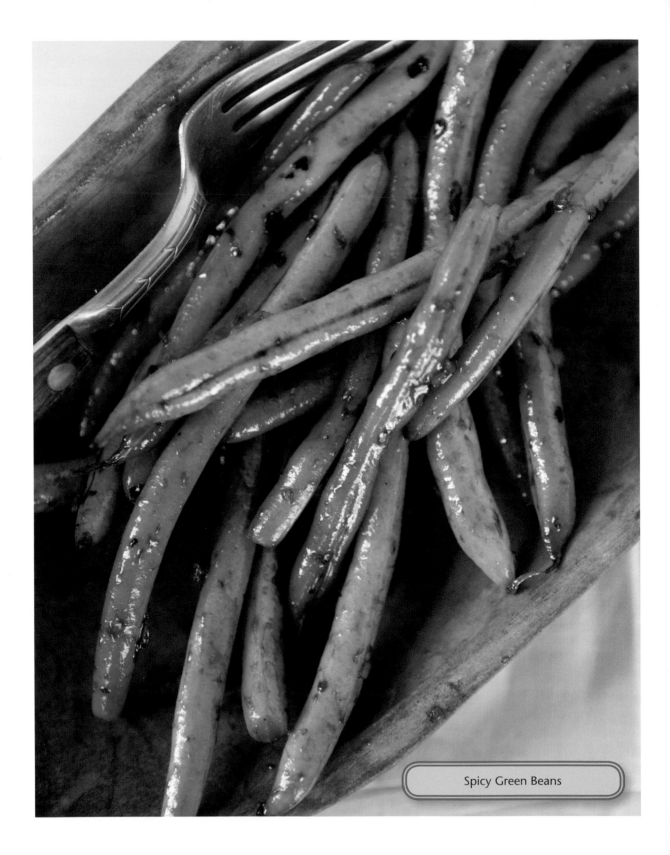

Spicy Green Beans

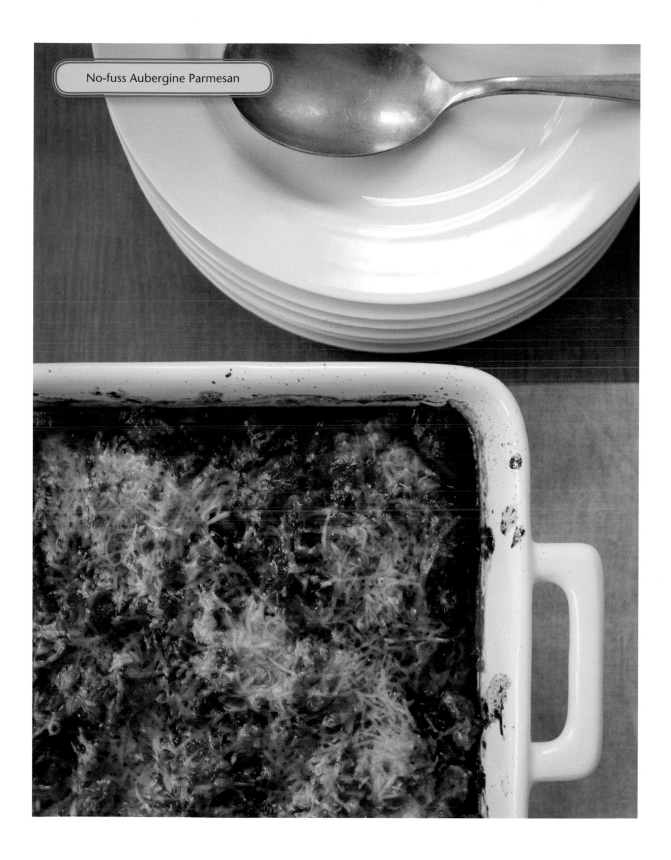

No-fuss Aubergine Parmesan

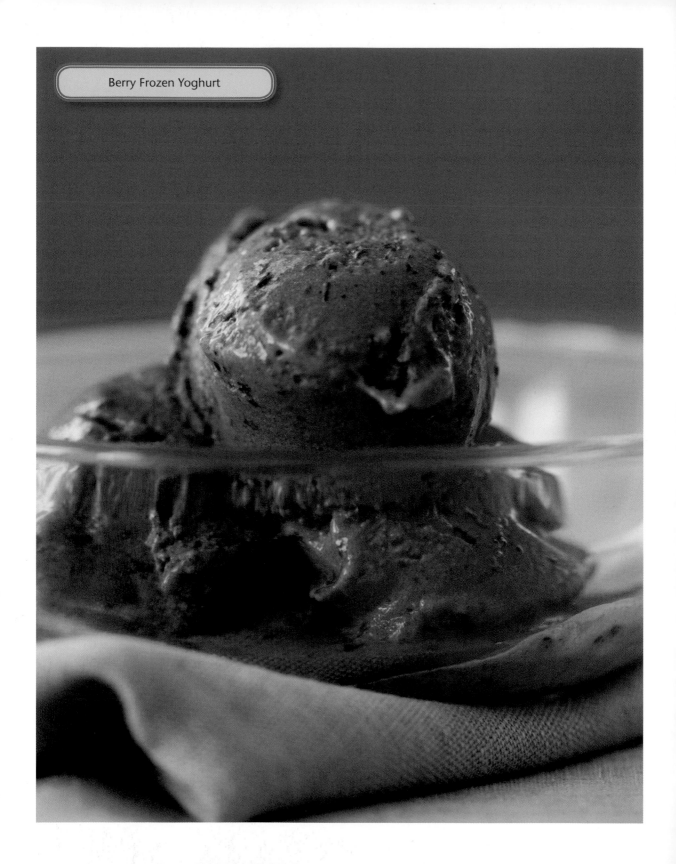

Berry Frozen Yoghurt

Chocolatey Frozen Yoghurt

If you love chocolate ice cream, you'll love this recipe. It will definitely keep you from plunging headlong into a tub of your favorite chocolate ice cream.

INGREDIENTS
    350 g/12 oz Greek 2% yogurt
    1 tablespoon low-fat buttermilk
    1 tablespoon agave nectar
    2 teaspoons unsweetened cocoa
    4 tablespoons sugar-free hot chocolate mix
    ½ teaspoon instant espresso powder
    ½ teaspoon vanilla extract

DIRECTIONS
1. Combine all the ingredients. Mix well using a whisk.

2. Refrigerate for a few hours until the mixture is very cold.

3. Freeze in an ice-cream machine according to the manufacturer's instructions.

YIELD: 2 servings

Spiced Plum Soup

Soup's on in the form of a sweet dessert. Soup is filling, so save room for this!

INGREDIENTS
    450 g/1 lb red or black plums, stoned and coarsely chopped
    350 ml/12 fl oz water
    1½ tablespoons Truvia
    1½ teaspoons ground cinnamon
    ¼ teaspoon ground cloves
    ½ cup natural low-fat Greek yoghurt
    Chopped mint leaves, optional

DIRECTIONS
1. Combine the plums, water, Truvia, cinnamon and cloves in a medium saucepan. Bring to a simmer over a medium heat, stirring occasionally. Cover, reduce the heat to low, and simmer very slowly until the plums have softened, for about 15 minutes, stirring occasionally.

2. Cool for 10 minutes. Transfer the entire contents of the saucepan to a large blender or food processor. Add the yoghurt, cover and process until smooth. Chill for at least 1 hour before serving. Garnish with chopped mint leaves, if desired.

YIELD: 4 servings

> **TIP:** If you like a kick in your sweet desserts, the soup is nice with ⅛ teaspoon cayenne added with the cinnamon and cloves. Store the soup, covered, in the fridge for up to 4 days.

17 Sample Cycle 1 Menus

Here are examples of how you can create your daily menu using the Accelerate Cycle recipes.

Day 1

Breakfast

- ☐ 1 serving *Snappy Eggs*
- ☐ ½ grapefruit or other fresh fruit
- ☐ 1 cup green tea

Lunch

- ☐ 1 serving *California Tuna Salad*
- ☐ 1 cup green tea

Dinner

- ☐ 1 serving *Tandoori Chicken Breasts*
- ☐ 1 cup green tea

Snack

- ☐ 175 g/6 oz non-fat yoghurt mixed with 1 or 2 tablespoons sugar-free jam
- ☐ 1 serving Cycle 1 fruit

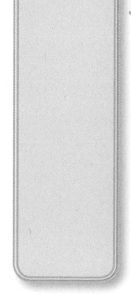

Breakfast

☐ 1 serving *Peach Melba Smoothie*

☐ 1 cup green tea

Lunch

☐ 1 serving *Super Salad*

☐ 1 cup green tea

Dinner

☐ 1 serving *Blackened Mahi-Mahi* with liberal amounts of any Cycle 1 vegetables, steamed or raw

☐ 1 cup green tea

Snack

☐ 175 g/6 oz sugar-free fruit-flavoured yoghurt, or 225 g/8 oz natural low-fat yogurt, sweetened with Truvia or a tablespoon of sugar-free fruit jam

☐ 1 serving fruit

Day 3

Breakfast

- ☐ 1 serving *Mushroom Spinach Frittata*
- ☐ ½ grapefruit or other fresh fruit in season
- ☐ 1 cup green tea

Lunch

- ☐ 1 large bowl *Chicken-Vegetable Soup*
- ☐ 1 cup green tea

Dinner

- ☐ Plenty of roast turkey breast or turkey fillet, steamed carrots and steamed asparagus.
- ☐ 1 cup green tea

Snack

- ☐ 175 g/6 oz natural non-fat yoghurt, sweetened with Truvia or a tablespoon of sugar-free fruit jam
- ☐ 1 serving *Kefir Smoothie*

Day 4

Breakfast

☐ 1 serving *Kefir Smoothie*

☐ 1 cup green tea

Lunch

☐ 1 serving *Turkey Picadillo Lettuce Wraps*

Dinner

☐ 1 serving *No-fuss Aubergine Parmesan*

☐ 1 cup green tea

Snack

☐ 175 g/6 oz natural non-fat yoghurt with a sliced fresh peach or other fruit in season

☐ 1 cup green tea

Day 5

Breakfast

- ☐ 2 scrambled egg whites
- ☐ ½ grapefruit or other fresh fruit in season
- ☐ 1 cup green tea

Lunch

- ☐ 1 serving *Super Salad*
- ☐ 1 cup green tea

Dinner

- ☐ 1 serving *Stir-Fried Chicken and Cucumbers*
- ☐ 1 cup green tea

Snacks

- ☐ 125 g/4½ oz fresh berries
- ☐ 175 g/6 oz natural non-fat yoghurt, sweetened with Truvia or a tablespoon of sugar-free fruit jam

NOTES

Breakfast

☐ 175 g/6 oz non-fat yoghurt, mixed with 125 g/4½ oz fresh berries or other fruit on the list. You may sweeten with 1 sachet of Truvia or a tablespoon of sugar-free fruit jam.

☐ 1 cup green tea

Lunch

☐ Griddled, then grilled chicken breast with tossed salad drizzled with 1 tablespoon olive or linseed oil and 2 tablespoons balsamic vinegar

☐ 1 cup green tea

Dinner

☐ 1 serving *Curried Poached Halibut*

☐ 1 cup green tea

Snacks

☐ 1 serving *Spiced Plum Soup*

☐ 2nd probiotic serving of your choice

Day 7

Breakfast

☐ 1 serving *Snappy Eggs*

☐ 1 apple or 125 g/4½ oz fresh berries

☐ 1 cup green tea

Lunch

☐ 1 serving *Super Salad*

☐ 1 cup green tea

Dinner

☐ 1 serving *Bavarian Chicken Breasts*

☐ 1 cup green tea

Snacks

☐ 2nd fruit serving + 1 probiotic serving of your choice

☐ 2nd probiotic serving of your choice

Day 8

Breakfast

☐ 175 g/6 oz non-fat yoghurt, mixed with 125 g/4½ oz fresh berries or other fruit on the list. You may sweeten with 1 sachet of Truvia or a tablespoon of sugar-free fruit jam.

☐ 1 cup green tea

Lunch

☐ 1 serving *Lemon-Pepper Salmon Salad in Tomato Cups*

☐ 1 cup green tea

Dinner

☐ Turkey burgers (made with lean turkey mince)

☐ Steamed Cycle 1 vegetables

☐ Side salad drizzled with drizzled with 1 tablespoon olive or linseed oil, mixed with 2 tablespoons balsamic vinegar and seasonings

☐ 1 cup green tea

Snack

☐ 1 serving *Berry Frozen Yoghurt*

Day 9

Breakfast

- ☐ 1 serving *Greek Egg Scramble*
- ☐ 1 fresh orange
- ☐ 1 cup green tea

Lunch

- ☐ 1 serving *Griddled Tuna Niçoise Salad*
- ☐ 1 cup green tea

Dinner

- ☐ Griddled chicken breast marinated in fat-free Italian dressing, then grilled
- ☐ Steamed Cycle 1 vegetables
- ☐ 1 cup green tea

Snacks

- ☐ *Peach Melba Smoothie*
- ☐ 175 g/6 oz non-fat yoghurt sweetened with Truvia or sugar-free fruit jam

Breakfast

- ☐ 115 g/4 oz natural cottage cheese
- ☐ 1 medium pear, sliced
- ☐ 1 cup green tea

Lunch

- ☐ 1 *Balsamic Artichoke*, served with non-fat salad dressing
- ☐ 1 serving *Green Tea-spiked Apple Sauce*
- ☐ 1 cup green tea

Dinner

- ☐ 1 serving *Oven-barbecued Chicken*
- ☐ Side salad drizzled with 1 tablespoon olive or linseed oil, mixed with 2 tablespoons balsamic vinegar and seasonings
- ☐ 1 cup green tea

Snacks

- ☐ 2nd probiotic serving
- ☐ Raw cut-up veggies

Day 11

Breakfast

- ☐ 1 serving *Yoghurt Fruitshake*
- ☐ 1 cup green tea

Lunch

- ☐ 1 serving *Super Salad*
- ☐ 1 cup green tea

Dinner

- ☐ Turkey burgers (made with lean turkey mince)
- ☐ 1 serving *Oven-roasted Cauliflower and Broccoli*
- ☐ 1 cup green tea

Snacks

- ☐ 1 serving *Berry Frozen Yoghurt*

NOTES

Breakfast

- ☐ 2 hard-boiled or poached eggs
- ☐ ½ grapefruit or other fresh fruit
- ☐ 1 cup green tea

Lunch

- ☐ Baked or grilled chicken breast
- ☐ Tomatoes, sliced or stewed
- ☐ 1 cup green tea

Dinner

- ☐ 1 serving *Baked Tilapia Parcels*
- ☐ 1 cup green tea

Snacks

- ☐ 1 serving *Kefir Smoothie*
- ☐ 1 serving *Berry Frozen Yoghurt*

Day 13

Breakfast

☐ 1 serving *Peach Melba Smoothie*

☐ 1 cup green tea

Lunch

☐ 1 serving *California Tuna Salad*

☐ 1 cup green tea

Dinner

☐ Plenty of roast turkey or chicken

☐ 1 serving *Spicy Green Beans*

☐ 1 cup green tea

Snacks

☐ 2nd fruit serving

☐ 1 serving *Berry Frozen Yoghurt*

Day 14

Breakfast

☐ 1 serving of *Mushroom Spinach Frittata*

☐ 1 apple or 125 g/4½ oz fresh berries

☐ 1 cup green tea

Lunch

☐ 1 large bowl *Chicken-Vegetable Soup*

☐ 1 cup green tea

Dinner

☐ 1 serving *Tandoori Chicken Breasts*

☐ 1 cup green tea

Snacks

☐ 1 medium pear or other fruit

☐ 175 g/6 oz non-fat yoghurt sweetened with Truvia or sugar-free fruit jam

Day 15

Breakfast

- ☐ 115 g/4 oz natural cottage cheese
- ☐ 1 medium pear, sliced
- ☐ 1 cup green tea

Lunch

- ☐ 1 serving *No-fuss Aubergine Parmesan*
- ☐ 1 cup green tea

Dinner

- ☐ 1 serving *Low-carb Primavera Delight*
- ☐ 1 cup green tea

Snacks

- ☐ 2nd fruit serving
- ☐ 1 serving *Berry Frozen Yoghurt*

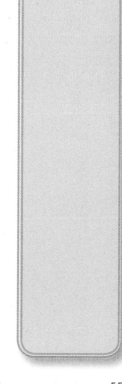

NOTES

Day 16

Breakfast

- ☐ 1 serving *Spanish Omelette*
- ☐ ½ grapefruit or 1 medium orange
- ☐ 1 cup green tea

Lunch

- ☐ 1 serving *Creamy Smoked Salmon Rolls*
- ☐ 1 cup green tea

Dinner

- ☐ Plenty of roast turkey breast or turkey fillet, steamed carrots and steamed asparagus.
- ☐ 1 cup green tea

Snacks

- ☐ 1 piece fresh fruit
- ☐ 175 g/6 oz non-fat yoghurt sweetened with Truvia or sugar-free fruit jam

Day 17

Breakfast

☐ 1 serving *Yoghurt Fruitshake*

☐ 1 cup green tea

Lunch

☐ 1 serving *Super Salad*

☐ 1 cup green tea

Dinner

☐ 1 serving *Baked Tilapia Parcels*

☐ 1 cup green tea

Snacks

☐ 1 medium apple

☐ 1 serving *Berry Frozen Yoghurt*

RECIPES

Cycle 2 – Activate

> **GOAL:** To reset your metabolism through a strategy that involves increasing and decreasing your caloric consumption to stimulate fat-burning and to help prevent plateaus.

Dr Mike's Power Cookie

My experience in medicine convinced me that the best approach to both snacks and meals is to present a varied diet with numerous choices, which is why I give you cookies! Yes, imagine being able to eat cookies on a diet. Well, now you can. I keep a large wide-mouthed jar full of these nutritious cookies. They are high in protein, very satisfying and have sweet-tooth appeal. Include these in your plan, and you'll feel and look like one smart cookie.

INGREDIENTS

85 g/3 oz unsweetened apple sauce
2 tablespoons almond paste
1 tablespoon linseed oil
10 sachets of Truvia
60 ml/2 fl oz agave nectar
1 medium egg
½ teaspoon vanilla essence
90 g/3¼ oz wholemeal flour
½ teaspoon bicarbonate of soda
1 teaspoon cinnamon
½ teaspoon salt
¼ teaspoon black pepper
75 g/2½ oz vanilla whey powder
185 g/6½ oz porridge oats
150 g/5½ oz dried cherries
200 g/7 oz flaked almonds
Non-stick cooking spray

DIRECTIONS

1. Heat oven to Gas Mark 4/180°C/fan oven 160°C. Beat together the apple sauce, almond paste, linseed oil, Truvia and agave nectar. Beat in the egg and vanilla. Mix well. Add the flour, bicarbonate of soda, cinnamon, salt, pepper and whey powder. Beat thoroughly. Stir in the oats, cherries and almonds. Mix well.

(continued on next page)

Dr Mike's Power Cookie (*cont.*)

2. Spray a baking tray with non-stick cooking spray. Divide the mixture into 18 balls using a large spoon and place them on the baking tray. Flatten the balls with the back of a spoon. Bake for 16 to 18 minutes or until soft and brown. Remove from oven. Cool and store in a covered container.

YIELD: 18 cookies

> TIP: Each cookie supplies 128 calories and can be enjoyed on the Activate, Achieve and Arrive cycles for breakfast or as a snack. Each cookie counts as 1 protein and 1 natural starch.

Eggs, Salmon and Onions

Call me a little crazy, but I dig fish first thing in the morning, if it's salmon, that is. There's just nothing better than good smoked salmon. In the USA , it is served with bagels, spread with cream cheese. Here, it's paired with eggs, and what a great match it is. You won't miss the bagel.

INGREDIENTS

    2 teaspoons olive oil
    1 small white onion, finely chopped
    2 medium eggs
    2 medium egg whites
    115 g/4 oz smoked salmon, chopped
    ½ teaspoon black pepper

DIRECTIONS

1. Heat the oil in a large non-stick frying pan over a medium heat. Add the onion. Cook, stirring often, until softened and lightly browned, for about 6 minutes.

2. Whisk the eggs and egg whites in a large bowl until well blended. Pour into the pan, then reduce the heat to low. Stir until curds begin to form. Add the salmon and pepper and continue stirring until the eggs are set, for about 1 minute.

YIELD: 2 servings (can be doubled)

> **TIP:** You can substitute smoked trout or smoked mackerel for salmon in this recipe.

Weekend Morning Polenta Bake

I'm particularly proud of this dish, and my vegetarian friends love it. The bake has everything you need for a good hearty breakfast: wholegrains, protein, veggies and fruit.

INGREDIENTS

Non-stick cooking spray

85 g/3 oz quick-cooking polenta

175 g/6 oz vegetarian sausages, crumbled, or sausage-flavoured textured soya protein such as Quorn

4 medium spring onions, finely chopped

1 tablespoon Worcestershire sauce

1 tablespoon finely chopped fresh oregano leaves or 1 teaspoon dried oregano

¼ teaspoon garlic powder

1 tart green apple, peeled and coarsely grated

115 g/4 oz fat-free Cheddar or Parmesan cheese, grated

1 medium egg

1medium egg white

DIRECTIONS

1. Bring 450 ml/16 fl oz water to a boil in a large saucepan over a high heat. Stir in the polenta, reduce the heat and simmer, stirring almost constantly, until thick, for about 4 minutes.

2. Remove the pan from the heat. Stir in the sausage, spring onions, Worcestershire sauce, oregano and garlic powder. Set aside for 10 minutes.

3. Meanwhile, position a shelf in the centre of the oven; preheat to Gas Mark 5/190°C/fan oven 170°C. Lightly spray the inside of a 20-cm/8-inch square baking tin with non-stick cooking spray.

4. Stir the apple and cheese into the polenta. Pour and spread this mixture into the prepared baking tin.

5. Bake until puffed, brown and set, for about 25 minutes. Cool for 5 minutes before cutting into squares.

YIELD: 4 servings

Super Strawberry Smoothie

If you're not into smoothies for breakfast, we need to talk. These blended drinks are the quickest breakfasts you can imagine, as well as being a super-healthy way to start the day. I like making mine with yoghurt. In addition to being a good source of protein and calcium, its low levels of lactose are easy for everyone to tolerate. And remember, probiotics like yoghurt and kefir are fat-burners par excellence.

INGREDIENTS

150 g/5 oz frozen strawberries, partially thawed

175 g/6 oz sugar-free low-fat strawberry yoghurt

60 ml/2 fl oz plain, low-fat kefir

1 tablespoon oat bran

¼ teaspoon grated nutmeg

2 ice cubes

DIRECTIONS

Place all the ingredients in a blender. Cover and blend until smooth, pulsing occasionally to make sure everything is well blended, and scraping down the inside of the container once or twice – turn the blender off when you do this.

YIELD: 1 serving

TIP: If the berries are really hard, it helps to shake the blender a bit.

Italian Prawn and White Bean Salad

When you see prawns as an ingredient in many recipes, it's usually a good sign because the recipes are probably low in calories and high in fat-burning protein. Another ingredient is white beans, which provide filling, satisfying fibre. This prawn salad balances taste, texture and nutrition to great effect. So there you have it: savoury, smooth and tangy. And healthy. This is an easy salad to make, too.

INGREDIENTS
225 g/8 oz raw medium prawns, peeled and de-veined
400 g/14 oz canned cannellini beans, drained and rinsed
3 medium celery sticks, finely chopped
½ small red onion, finely chopped
60 ml/2 fl oz low-fat, sugar-free creamy Italian dressing

DIRECTIONS
1. Bring a large saucepan of water to the boil. Add the prawns. Cook until pink and firm, for about 3 minutes. Drain in a colander. Rinse with cool tap water to stop the cooking. Drain thoroughly by shaking the colander.

2. Chop the prawns on a chopping board, then place in a serving bowl. Add the beans, celery, onion and dressing, and stir well.

YIELD: 2 servings (can be doubled)

> **TIP:** To save time, use cooked, peeled and deveined prawns. You can stir everything together in minutes.

Crab Tabouleh

Tabouleh *is a traditional Middle Eastern salad featuring vegetables and bulgar wheat. This recipe adds crab, which enhances the other ingredients remarkably well.*

INGREDIENTS

75 g/2½ oz quick-cooking bulgar
175 g/6 oz crabmeat, picked over for bits of shell and cartilage
250 g/9 oz canned chickpeas, drained and rinsed
85 g/3 oz frozen sweetcorn, thawed
2 medium spring onions, thinly sliced
1 roasted red pepper, chopped
60 ml/2 fl oz low-fat, sugar-free balsamic vinaigrette

DIRECTIONS

1. Place the bulgar in a large, heat-proof mixing bowl. Pour 450 ml/16 fl oz boiling water over the bulgar and set aside until the water has been absorbed, for about 20 minutes.

2. Stir in the crabmeat, chickpeas, sweetcorn, spring onions, red pepper and vinaigrette.

YIELD: 2 servings (can be doubled)

TIP: Canned crabmeat is available in most supermarkets. Some supermarkets sell dressed crab, or purchase crabmeat from your fishmonger. However, even ready-prepared crabmeat needs to be put on a plate or chopping board and picked over in case there are any fragments of bone or shell.

Warm Curried Quinoa Salad

Quinoa is lower in carbohydrates than most grains and is an excellent source of protein. It's highly nutritious, very tasty, easy to prepare and great if you're gluten intolerant. Featuring roasted red peppers, onions, garlic and ginger, and more, in a taste-bud-bursting dressing, this salad is fantastic.

INGREDIENTS

85 g/3 oz beige or red quinoa

Non-stick cooking spray

1 small white onion, chopped

1 tablespoon peeled, finely chopped fresh root ginger or ready-prepared finely chopped root ginger

1 medium garlic clove, finely chopped, or 1 teaspoon ready-prepared finely chopped garlic

1 tablespoon curry powder

¼ teaspoon salt

225 g/8 oz cabbage, coarsely grated

1½ tablespoons apple-cider vinegar

1 medium sweet apple, such as Gala or Fuji, peeled and coarsely grated

3 tablespoons low-fat, sugar-free bottled ranch dressing

DIRECTIONS

1. Bring 250 ml/8 fl oz water to the boil in a medium saucepan over a high heat. Stir in the quinoa. Reduce the heat to low and cook until the water has been absorbed and the quinoa is tender, for about 12 minutes.

2. Spray a large non-stick frying pan with non-stick cooking spray. Set over a medium heat for 1 minute, then add the onion, ginger and garlic. Cook, stirring often, until softened, for about 3 minutes. Stir in the curry powder and salt and cook until fragrant, for about 20 seconds.

3. Add the cabbage and vinegar. Scrape up any browned bits on the base of the pan as the vinegar comes to a boil. Cover, reduce the

heat to low, and cook until the cabbage is tender, for about 10 minutes.

4. Remove the pan from the heat. Stir in the apple, cooked quinoa and dressing.

YIELD: 2 servings

> **TIP:** For an on-the-go lunch, make ahead and warm in the microwave.
>
> Some quinoa has a bitter chemical compound – *saponin* – still on the seeds. Most have been washed to remove this compound. However, if you buy quinoa in bulk or inexpensive packaging in international markets, you probably should rinse the quinoa in a colander before cooking to remove this compound.

Smoked Turkey and Lentil Salad

Diets are synonymous with salads. Instead of just tossing together some lettuce, celery, tomato and a splatter of dressing, why not try new flavour combinations? You can turn a salad into something exceptional with just a few interesting ingredients, such as lentils, a staple of vegetarians and the popular Mediterranean diet. I love lentils in any form; they're rich in protein, vitamin B and iron, and taste great with smoked turkey and spices here.

INGREDIENTS

150 g/5 oz dried green lentils

175 g/6 oz sandwich-style smoked turkey, diced

3 medium celery sticks, finely chopped

1 large carrot, coarsely grated

60 ml/2 fl oz low-fat, sugar-free, bottled creamy Italian vinaigrette

2 teaspoons fresh thyme leaves or ½ teaspoon dried thyme

½ teaspoon ground black pepper

DIRECTIONS

1. Fill a large saucepan about two-thirds full with water and bring to the boil over a high heat. Add the lentils and reduce the heat to low. Simmer until tender, for about 15 minutes. Drain the lentils in a colander. Rinse with cool tap water to stop the cooking. Drain thoroughly, shaking the colander.

2. Pour the lentils into a large bowl. Stir in the turkey, celery, carrot, dressing, thyme and pepper.

YIELD: 2 servings

Falafel Salad

Falafel is made from chickpeas, bulgar wheat and spices. It is high in fibre and protein, and has no cholesterol. Added to a salad, it may make the perfect vegetarian meal.

INGREDIENTS

75 g/2½ oz quick-cooking bulgar
250 g/9 oz canned chickpeas, drained and rinsed
15 g/½ oz parsley leaves
2 medium spring onions, thinly sliced
1 medium garlic clove, peeled
1 medium egg white
1 teaspoon baking powder
1 teaspoon ground cumin
½ teaspoon cinnamon
½ teaspoon salt
½ teaspoon black pepper
1 tablespoon olive oil
250 g/9 oz mixed salad leaves
1 large tomato, chopped
1 medium cucumber, peeled and chopped
125 ml/4 fl oz low-fat, sugar-free bottled ranch dressing

DIRECTIONS

1. Put the bulgar in a large, heat-proof bowl. Pour 250 ml/8 fl oz boiling water over the bulgar. Set aside until the water has been absorbed, for about 30 minutes.

2. Scrape the bulgar into a large food processor fitted with a chopping blade. Add the chickpeas, parsley, spring onions, garlic, egg white, baking powder, cumin, cinnamon, salt, and pepper. Cover and blend until the mixture becomes a grainy paste, scraping

(continued on next page)

Falafel Salad (*cont.*)

down the inside of the canister once or twice – turn the machine off when you do this.

3. Heat the oil in a large non-stick frying pan over a medium heat. With wet hands, pat the paste into four patties, slipping them one by one into the pan. Cook until brown and fairly dry on one side, for about 4 minutes. Turn the patties and continue cooking until brown and set, for about 4 more minutes. Transfer to a chopping board.

4. Mix the salad leaves, tomato, cucumber and dressing in a large bowl. Divide among four plates. Top with a falafel.

YIELD: 4 servings

> **TIP:** For an on-the-go lunch, keep the salad dressing separate from the leaves until you're ready to eat. The cooked falafel patties freeze well. Once thoroughly cooled, wrap in cling film and store in the freezer for up to 3 months. Warm in a dry frying pan over a medium heat for a few minutes, turning once; or on a baking tray in a preheated oven Gas Mark 4/180°C/fan oven 160°C for 10 minutes.

Cantonese Stir-fried Prawns

I thought I'd just go ahead and get the preachy eat-more-veggies sermon out of the way now. You'll certainly do that with this recipe. It's very similar to the prawns-with-mange-tout dish you find in many Cantonese restaurants. But there are even more veggies in this version.

INGREDIENTS

Non-stick cooking spray

2 medium spring onions, finely chopped

1 tablespoon peeled, finely chopped, fresh root ginger or ready-prepared finely chopped root ginger

1 medium garlic clove, finely chopped, or 1 teaspoon ready-prepared finely chopped garlic

175 g/6 oz chestnut or white button mushrooms, thinly sliced

450 g/1 lb raw medium prawns, peeled and de-veined

175 g/6 oz mange tout, trimmed

400 g/14 oz baby corn, drained and rinsed if canned

2 tablespoons fat-free, low-sodium chicken stock

1 tablespoon light soy sauce

1 tablespoon oyster sauce, optional

DIRECTIONS

1. Spray a large wok, preferably non-stick, with non-stick cooking spray. Set it over a high heat until just smoking, for about 3 minutes. Add the spring onions, ginger and garlic. Toss and stir over the heat until aromatic, for about 30 seconds.

2. Add the mushrooms and stir-fry for 1 minute. Add the prawns and continue tossing and stirring over the heat for 1 minute.

3. Add the mange tout and baby corn. Stir-fry for 1 minute. Pour in the stock and keep stir-frying until the wok is almost dry, for about another minute. Finally, add the soy sauce and the oyster sauce, if using. Toss a few times before serving.

YIELD: 4 servings

(continued on next page)

Cantonese Stir-fried Prawns (*cont.*)

TIPS: Have bags of frozen prawns to hand in Cycle 2. To thaw more quickly, place in a bowl, cover with water and leave to stand for 10 minutes, changing the water once. Oyster sauce is an option here because it's so very Cantonese. It's available in the Oriental aisle of most supermarkets.

Roasted Prawns and Broccoli

No time to cook? Well, if you can spare just 12 minutes, here's the dinner for you. It's a super-quick one-pot meal that you can serve up in no time.

INGREDIENTS

680 g/1 lb 8 oz frozen broccoli florets, thawed

450 g/1 lb (about 30) raw medium prawns, peeled and de-veined

1 tablespoon olive oil

1 tablespoon lemon juice

2 medium garlic cloves, finely chopped, or 2 teaspoons ready-prepared finely chopped garlic

1 teaspoon finely grated lemon zest

½ teaspoon dried chilli flakes

½ teaspoon salt

DIRECTIONS

1. Position a shelf in the centre of the oven; preheat the oven to Gas Mark 7/220°C/fan oven 200°C.

2. Mix all the ingredients in a large roasting tin or the grill pan. Bake until the prawns are pink and firm, for about 12 minutes, tossing once or twice.

YIELD: 4 servings

> **TIP:** You can find already peeled and de-veined prawns at almost every supermarket. Just don't use cooked prawns.

Stewed Mussels

Many people are shy of mussels, but I love them no matter how they're prepared. Cooked mussels, grilled mussels, fried mussels and now stewed mussels: a meal of mussels is the meal for me. But no mussel recipe has ever tasted so good to me as this one. Mussels are low in fat, high in omega 3, and packed with high levels of daily requirements for zinc, vitamin C and iron.

INGREDIENTS

1 medium white onion, chopped

4 medium celery sticks, finely chopped

800 g/1 lb 12 oz canned chopped tomatoes

400 g/14 oz artichoke-heart quarters bottled in water, drained and rinsed

2 tablespoons finely chopped fresh oregano leaves or 2 teaspoons dried oregano

2 tablespoons fresh thyme leaves or 2 teaspoons dried thyme

½ teaspoon dried chilli flakes, optional

1.8 kg/4 lb mussels, cleaned and debearded

DIRECTIONS

1. Combine the onion, celery, tomatoes, artichokes, oregano, thyme, and chilli flakes, if using, in a very large pan. Bring to the boil over a high heat. Reduce the heat to low, cover and simmer slowly for 10 minutes.

2. Stir in the mussels. Raise the heat to medium, cover and continue cooking until the mussels open, for about 12 minutes. Pour the contents of the pot into a large serving bowl. Discard any mussels that do not open.

YIELD: 4 servings

TIPS: Ask for a small bag of ice from the supermarket or fishmonger to keep mussels cool, particularly on a warm day. Place them in a large bowl and refrigerate. To debeard mussels, pull the wiry threads from their shells along the seam until they snap free. Rinse to remove any sand. Do not cook any mussels that are open and refuse to shut when tapped. Cook mussels on the same day you buy them.

Easy Chicken Posole

You'll go crazy over this chicken posole, a hearty stew with an American Southwestern attitude, based on green chilli peppers, cumin and garlic. This dish, which uses canned hominy, available from online Mexican food specialists, takes a fraction of the time needed for regular posole.

INGREDIENTS

Non-stick cooking spray

1 medium white onion, chopped

1 medium red pepper, deseeeded and chopped

1 medium garlic clove, finely chopped, or 1 teaspoon ready-prepared finely chopped garlic

450 g/1 lb boneless skinless chicken breasts, cut into 2.5-cm/1-inch pieces

850 g/1 lb 14 oz canned hominy, drained and rinsed

115 g/4 oz canned chopped green chillies, mild or hot

2 teaspoons dried oregano

1 teaspoon ground cumin

350 ml/12 fl oz fat-free, low-sodium chicken stock

55 g/2 oz fat-free soured cream, optional

10 g/¼ oz fresh coriander leaves, finely chopped

Lime wedges, optional

DIRECTIONS

1. Spray a large saucepan with non-stick cooking spray and set the pan over a medium heat for 1 minute. Add the onion, red pepper and garlic and cook, stirring often, until softened, for about 3 minutes.

2. Stir in the chicken breasts. Continue cooking, stirring often, until the chicken loses its raw, pink colour, for about 5 minutes.

3. Add the hominy, chillies, oregano and cumin; stir for 1 minute. Pour in the stock; raise the heat to high and stir occasionally as the mixture comes to the boil. Cover, reduce the heat to low and simmer for 20 minutes. Ladle into serving bowls; top each with 1 tablespoon soured cream, if using, and 1 tablespoon chopped

fresh coriander leaves. Serve with lime wedges on the side to squeeze into the stew, if using.

YIELD: 4 servings

> **TIP:** To save time, you can use frozen chopped onions in place of a chopped onion. One medium white onion = 115 g/4 oz frozen chopped onion. No need to thaw frozen chopped onions. Use them straight from the freezer. If you can't find hominy, substitute 750 g/1 lb 10 oz pearl barley, following the packet instructions for cooking.

Turkey and Bulgar Meatloaf

When it's cold, snowy or rainy outside, what else is there to do but snuggle up with a plate of comfort food? The problem is that traditionally means something loaded with fat and calories, a dish that can latch right on to your hips and thighs. This recipe reduces all the bad stuff without being a traitor to tradition. Using turkey mince and bulgar instead of high-carb bread crumbs helps you keep a careful watch over your diet. Dig in, and you'll get a hefty dose of nutrition. This no-fuss recipe will have your loved ones saying, "Make that again, please!"

INGREDIENTS

75 g/2½ oz quick-cooking bulgar

Non-stick cooking spray

450 g/1 lb lean turkey mince

1 medium egg white

1 tablespoon Dijon mustard

1½ teaspoons salt-free Italian spice or seasoning blend

½ teaspoon salt

½ teaspoon ground black pepper

DIRECTIONS

1. Place the bulgar in a large blender, cover and blend until finely ground, for about 1 minute. Tip the ground bulgar into a heat-proof bowl, pour over 175 ml/6 fl oz boiling water, cover and set aside to cool for about 30 minutes.

2. Position a shelf in the centre of the oven and preheat the oven to Gas Mark 4/180°C/fan oven 160°C. Spray a 23- x 33-cm/9- x 13-inch ovenproof dish lightly with non-stick cooking spray.

3. Pour the bulgar into a large bowl and fluff with a fork. Mix in the turkey mince, egg white, mustard, spice blend, salt and pepper. Form the mixture into an oval mound and set in a baking tin.

4. Bake until browned and cooked through for about 50 minutes. Cool for 5 minutes before slicing.

YIELD: 4 servings

TIP: Want to be fancy? Spread the top of the unbaked meatloaf with 2 teaspoons Dijon mustard, sugar-free barbecue sauce, Worcestershire sauce, or sugar-free tomato ketchup.

Fast and Easy Chilli

If you take a look at the ingredients in many chilli recipes, you'll often find lots of fattening ingredients, like fatty cuts of meat or too much oil. That said, let's design the perfect chilli recipe. It has to be low-low fat and high in protein. It should be loaded with vitamins and minerals and have gobs of complex carbohydrates and fibre. And . . . and . . . oh, yeah. It should taste great. Know what we just designed? Fast and Easy Chilli.

INGREDIENTS

Non-stick cooking spray
450 g/1 lb lean steak mince
400 g/14 oz canned kidney beans, drained and rinsed
300 g/10½ oz ready-prepared mild or medium salsa
165 g/5¾ oz frozen sweetcorn niblets
2 tablespoons chilli powder
2 teaspoons lime juice
1 teaspoon ground cumin
55 g/2 oz fat-free soured cream, optional

DIRECTIONS

1. Spray a large saucepan with non-stick cooking spray. Set over a medium heat, then crumble in the steak mince. Cook, stirring often, until lightly browned, about 4 minutes.

2. Stir in the beans, salsa sauce, sweetcorn, chilli powder, lime juice and cumin. Bring to a full simmer. Cover, reduce the heat to low and cook for 15 minutes, stirring occasionally. Ladle into bowls and top each with 1 tablespoon fat-free soured cream, if using.

YIELD: 4 servings

TIP: The salsa I'd recommend is a medium heat sauce. Just steer clear of any fancy salsas such as chipotle. You want a plain, tomato-based salsa, not too hot (because it'll get hotter as it cooks and concentrates).

Slow-cooker Cuban Ropa Vieja

Ropa vieja *means 'old clothes', presumably because the shredded meat in this Cuban pot roast resembles rags. Don't let the name ruin your appetite. Just think of the old fat clothes you'll be shedding as you drop pounds and pounds of weight on the 17 Day Diet. Ropa vieja is one of my favourite dishes.*

INGREDIENTS

550 g/1 lb 4 oz top rump steak, trimmed

1 medium red onion, halved through the stem and thinly sliced

1 medium red pepper, deseeded and thinly sliced

1 medium green pepper, deseeded, and thinly sliced

2 medium garlic cloves, finely chopped, or 2 teaspoons ready-prepared garlic, finely chopped

1 teaspoon dried rosemary

1 teaspoon dried oregano

1 teaspoon ground cumin

½ teaspoon salt

½ teaspoon black pepper

350 ml/12 fl oz fat-free, low-sodium beef stock

2 tablespoons apple-cider vinegar

1 tablespoon tomato purée

Tabasco sauce, to taste

1 tablespoon fresh coriander leaves, optional

DIRECTIONS

1. Place the steak in the base of a 5- to 6-litre/8½- to 10-pint slow cooker. Place the onion, peppers, garlic, rosemary, oregano, cumin, salt and pepper over and around the meat. Whisk the stock, vinegar and tomato purée in a small bowl and pour over the meat and vegetables.

2. Cover and cook on low until the meat is tender enough to be shredded with a fork, for 8 to 10 hours. Use two forks to shred the beef into long, thin strips in the pot. If using, stir in some Tabasco sauce and fresh coriander before serving.

(continued on next page)

Slow-cooker Cuban Ropa Vieja (*cont.*)

YIELD: 4 servings

TIPS: To save time, use 300 g/10½ oz of frozen pepper strips in place of the two peppers. No need to thaw them. To make this dish on the hob, place the beef in a casserole dish, then add all the ingredients as directed in the recipe. Bring to a simmer over a medium-high heat, then reduce the heat to low, cover and simmer slowly until the meat is tender enough to be shredded with a fork, for about 2½ to 3 hours.

Tuscan Pork Tenderloin

I love one-pot meals like this one. Most of my food groups gather in one pan, and that means fewer dishes to wash! The tenderloin is the leanest cut of pork, and is as lean as a skinless chicken breast, and thus a great choice for Cycle 2.

INGREDIENTS

450 g/1 lb Brussels sprouts, trimmed

4 medium red-skinned potatoes, quartered

1 garlic head, broken into cloves, but not peeled

1 tablespoon olive oil

1 tablespoon salt-free Italian spice mix or seasoning blend

1 teaspoon finely grated lemon zest

½ teaspoon salt

550 g/1 lb 4 oz pork tenderloin

1 tablespoon lemon juice

DIRECTIONS

1. Position a shelf in the centre of the oven and preheat to Gas Mark 5/190°C/fan oven 170°C.

2. Place the Brussels sprouts, potatoes and garlic cloves in a large roasting tin or the grill pan. Toss with the olive oil, then roast for 25 minutes.

3. Meanwhile, mix the spice or seasoning blend, lemon zest and salt in a small bowl. Pat and smooth this mixture all over the tenderloin.

4. Move the vegetables to the sides of the tin without mounding them and set the tenderloin in the centre of the pan. Roast for another 20 minutes.

5. Turn the pork and toss the vegetables. Continue roasting until the meat is cooked through and the potatoes are tender for 15 to 20 additional minutes. Transfer the pork to a carving or chopping

(continued on next page)

Tuscan Pork Tenderloin (*cont.*)

board. Whilst the roasting tin is still hot, add the lemon juice and stir to scrape up any browned bits and coat the vegetables. Carve the pork into 1-cm-/½-inch-thick rounds to serve with the vegetables.

YIELD: 4 servings

TIP: Eat this by squeezing the warm garlic pulp out of the papery hulls and on to the vegetables and pork – it's a sort of roasted-garlic spread. You should probably wait about 10 minutes before serving so that the garlic is cool enough to be handled.

Brown Rice Biryani

Biryani is an Indian, Middle Eastern and Oriental dish made with rice and vegetables. It comes from the Persian word for roasted. You'll fall in love with this dish, especially after you see how little prep time is involved.

INGREDIENTS

900 g/2 lb frozen mixed vegetables

1 medium garlic clove, finely chopped, or 1 teaspoon ready-prepared finely chopped garlic

1 tablespoon ready-prepared finely chopped root ginger

250 ml/8 fl oz fat-free, low-sodium chicken stock

125 ml/4 fl oz natural, low-fat yoghurt

1½ tablespoons curry powder

15 g/½ oz fresh coriander leaves, finely chopped

1 tablespoon lemon juice

400 g/14 oz cooked brown basmati rice

Non-stick cooking spray

DIRECTIONS

1. Mix the vegetables, garlic, ginger, stock, yoghurt and curry powder in a large saucepan. Set over a medium heat and bring to a simmer, stirring occasionally. Cover, reduce the heat to low and cook for 10 minutes, stirring once in a while.

2. Meanwhile, position a shelf in the centre of the oven and preheat to Gas Mark 5/190°C/fan oven 170°C.

3. Stir the fresh coriander and lemon juice into the vegetable mixture. Pour into a 23-cm/9-inch square ovenproof dish. Spread the vegetables out evenly, then top with the cooked rice in a solid, fairly compact layer. Spray the top of the rice lightly with non-stick cooking spray and cover the dish tightly with kitchen foil.

(continued on next page)

SIDES, SNACKS AND DESSERTS

Brown Rice Biryani (*cont.*)

4. Bake for 20 minutes. Remove the foil and continue until the rice dries out and gets a little crispy, for about a further 10 minutes. Cool for 5 minutes before serving.

YIELD: 4 servings

Make Your Own Curry Blend
Mix these spices in a small bowl:
1 tablespoon ground coriander
1 tablespoon turmeric
1 tablespoon ground ginger
1 teaspoon ground fenugreek
1 teaspoon ground mace
1 teaspoon salt
½ teaspoon ground cloves
½ teaspoon ground cinnamon
½ teaspoon ground cumin
Up to ½ teaspoon cayenne
Use in place of ready-prepared curry powder; store in a sealed jar or small plastic container in a cool, dark place for up to 1 year.

TIP: Traditionally, a biryani is served by turning the whole dish out on to a big platter, the rice now on the bottom, the veggies on top. You can do that here – or just scoop out servings on to plates.

Easy Succotash

Succotash is an American sweetcorn-based dish with other veggies added in, including butter beans. In place of butter beans, we substituted high-protein edamame soya beans.

INGREDIENTS

  1 tablespoon olive oil

  1 medium white onion, chopped

  325 g/11½ oz frozen sweetcorn niblets

  280 g/10 oz frozen podded edamame soya beans

  1 medium red pepper, deseeded and cut into thin strips

  1 medium garlic clove, finely chopped, or 1 teaspoon ready-
      prepared finely chopped garlic

  1 tablespoon Cajun seasoning mix or spice blend

  125 ml/4 fl oz fat-free, low-sodium chicken stock

  1 tablespoon apple-cider vinegar

DIRECTIONS

1. Swirl the olive oil in a large, preferably non-stick, frying pan and set over a medium heat for 1 minute. Add the onion and cook until softened, for about 3 minutes, stirring occasionally.

2. Add the sweetcorn, edamame soya beans, red pepper and garlic and cook, stirring often, until hot, for about 4 minutes. Add the seasoning, then pour in the stock. Cook until liquid has almost evaporated, for about 7 minutes. Remove the pan from the heat and stir in the vinegar.

YIELD: 4 servings

> **TIPS:** To save time, use 150 g/5 oz frozen pepper strips instead of the whole pepper. You can store the remainder of the succotash in the fridge and use as a filling for an egg/egg white omelette or warm it up and use as a topping for scrambled eggs.

SIDES, SNACKS AND DESSERTS

Microwave Mashed Potatoes

Everyone loves mashed potatoes. The trouble is, you can't eat traditional mashed potatoes on most diets. Those delicious lumps of carbs can turn into unsightly lumps on your hips and thighs. Not so with this recipe! The addition of fat-free soured cream to delectable Maris Piper potatoes makes these mash potatoes taste like their fattening counterparts. Enjoy!

INGREDIENTS
4 medium Maris Piper potatoes

60 ml/2 fl oz fat-free, low-sodium chicken stock

2 tablespoons fat-free soured cream

1 tablespoon Dijon mustard

1 tablespoon finely chopped fresh or dried chives, optional

DIRECTIONS
1. Place the potatoes in a medium, microwave-safe bowl. Cover tightly with cling film and make a 2.5-cm/1-inch slit in the film. Alternatively, use a microwave-safe plastic bowl with a lid and open the small vent hole in the lid.

2. Microwave on high for 8 minutes. Remove the bowl from the microwave and set aside, covered, for 5 minutes.

3. Uncover and add the stock, soured cream, mustard and chives, if using. Mash with a potato masher or a hand-held electric mixer until fairly smooth. (Add a little more broth if you prefer looser mashed potatoes.)

YIELD: 4 servings

TIPS: The trick here is threefold: the potatoes must not be pricked or poked, the seal on the bowl must be tight and you can *only* use yellow-fleshed potatoes, like Maris Piper. Waxy potatoes don't have the right moisture/starch ratio to work in the microwave this way.

Butternut Squash Polenta

Polenta is the Italian version of a corn-based porridge. Cooking polenta used to be time-consuming, requiring constant stirring for almost an hour to make it smooth. Now, with quick-cooking polenta, it's a snap, and worth doing. Polenta pairs well with almost everything; here we've added butternut squash, a superfood packed with antioxidants.

INGREDIENTS

750 ml/1¼ pints fat-free, low-sodium chicken stock

550 g/1 lb 4 oz butternut squash, peeled, deseeded and diced, then cooked in boiling water for 5 minutes, drained and puréed

1 teaspoon ground cumin

½ teaspoon cinnamon

½ teaspoon salt

½ teaspoon black pepper

¼ teaspoon cayenne, optional

165 g/5¾ oz quick-cooking polenta

DIRECTIONS

1. Put the stock, puréed squash, cumin, cinnamon, salt, pepper and cayenne, if using, in a large saucepan. Set over a medium-high heat and whisk occasionally until the squash is smooth and the mixture comes to a simmer.

2. Reduce the heat to medium-low. Whisk in the polenta. Continue whisking until thick and creamy, about 3 minutes.

YIELD: 4 servings

> **TIPS:** A whisk is pretty crucial here to keep the polenta creamy. A wooden spoon will give you lumpier polenta, which is not the worst thing in the world but not the most desirable, either. As a variation, try adding 55 g/2 oz of finely grated fat-free cheese to the polenta, stirring it in at the end, after the pan is off the heat.

Mushroom Barley Sauté

Barley may be one of the oldest grains on earth. It was first used by the Egyptians ten thousand years ago, and taken to America by Christopher Columbus in 1494. Even so, it's not as popular as oats or rice. As a doctor, I'm pushing barley because it can help prevent lots of health conditions, ranging from unbalanced blood sugar levels to obesity to cardiovascular disease and cancer. Why is barley so beneficial? It's high in phytochemicals, which help ward off disease, and it is packed with soluble fibre, known to lower diabetes risk and reduce total blood cholesterol levels. Barley is truly a natural medicine.

INGREDIENTS

200 g/7 oz barley
Non-stick cooking spray
4 medium spring onions, thinly sliced
225 g/8 oz white button or chestnut mushrooms, thinly sliced
1 teaspoon dried thyme
½ teaspoon black pepper
1 tablespoon Worcestershire sauce

DIRECTIONS

1. Bring 750 ml/1¼ pint water to a boil in a saucepan. Add the barley, return to the boil, then reduce the heat to a simmer and cook for about 45–50 minutes, until the water is fully absorbed.

2. Spray a large frying pan with non-stick cooking spray and set it over a medium heat for 1 minute. Add the spring onions and mushrooms and cook, stirring often, until the mushrooms are tender, for 8 to 10 minutes.

3. Stir in the thyme and pepper and cook for 20 seconds. Add the cooked barley and the Worcestershire sauce and cook, stirring constantly, until heated through, for about 1 minute.

YIELD: 4 servings

TIP: The barley can be cooked in advance. Keep it in the fridge in a covered container for up to 3 days. Warm in a microwave for 1 minute on high before adding it to the frying pan.

Also, this can be used as a bed for the falafels in the Falafel Salad (page 71).

White Bean and Red Pepper Dip

You've got the munchies and just have to have some salt and something crunchy. Hold it – don't munch on crisps and dip! Be willing to push that junk aside. It's what you choose for a snack that makes a difference in your weight loss. Snacking on healthy foods can be a good and convenient way to satisfy your cravings, whilst giving your body a nutritional boost. Try this dip the next time you have a snack attack.

INGREDIENTS

400 g/14 oz canned cannellini beans, drained and rinsed

1 roasted red pepper, cut into 3 pieces

60 g/2¼ oz yoghurt cheese (see the recipe on page 18)

1 garlic clove, peeled

1 tablespoon lemon juice

½ teaspoon salt

½ teaspoon ground black pepper

DIRECTIONS

Place all the ingredients in a food processor fitted with the chopping blade and process until creamy, scraping down the inside of the bowl once or twice – turn the machine off when you do this.

YIELD: 4 servings

> **TIPS:** Serve with cut-up celery, cucumber rounds, baby carrots and broccoli florets. Take them to work in a separate container for a quick lunch.
>
> The dip stores well in a sealed container in the fridge for up to 3 days.

Spiced Edamame Soya Beans

It's no secret that to drop pounds or tackle our cholesterol, we have to watch fat and carbs, eat more veggies and turn cheesecake into a treat, not an everyday dessert. But have you ever wondered, whilst you're getting trim and healthy, how to eat to slow ageing and stay young? Beans are a great anti-ageing food, including edamame soya beans. This miracle veggie is loaded with heart-healthy folic acid and fibre to keep you slim. Plus, it's digested slowly and enters the bloodstream gradually, which minimises the spikes in blood sugar that can lead to cravings and weight gain. A few weeks from now, when you're slimmer and sexier, you'll be glad you put this version of edamame soya beans on your plate.

INGREDIENTS
450 g/1 lb frozen edamame soya beans in their pods

1 teaspoon salt

½ teaspoon ground coriander

½ teaspoon dried ginger

½ teaspoon dried chilli flakes, optional

DIRECTIONS
1. Bring a large pot of water to the boil over high heat. Add the edamame soya beans. Boil for 8 minutes. Drain in a colander. Lay some kitchen paper on your work surface and pour the edamame soya beans on top. Pat dry.

2. Place the cooked beans in a bowl and add the salt, coriander, ginger and chilli flakes, if using. Toss well.

YIELD: 4 servings

> **TIPS:** As you know, you don't eat the pods. You scrape the beans out through their pods with your teeth, getting some of the spice mixture as you do. You can also use 2½ teaspoons of the curry blend we made for the Brown Rice Biryani (page 88).

Mexican Chocolate Pudding

Chocolate is heavenly. Chocolate rules. Chocolate, my friends, is a terrible thing to shun on a diet. With this recipe, you can have your chocolate and eat it, too. It's a pudding made with high-protein, super-nutritious tofu. And if you think you don't like tofu, get over it. Tofu takes on whatever flavour it is paired with, including chocolate!

INGREDIENTS

350 g/12 oz silken extra-firm tofu

30 g/1 oz cocoa powder

3 tablespoons sugar-free chocolate-flavoured syrup

2 teaspoons Truvia

½ teaspoon almond extract

½ teaspoon cinnamon

¼ teaspoon or less cayenne, optional

DIRECTIONS

Place all the ingredients in a large food processor. Cover and process until smooth, for about 1 minute, scraping down the inside of the bowl at least once. Divide into four ramekins or small bowls and serve immediately or refrigerate.

YIELD: 4 servings

> **TIP:** It's important to get the silken extra-firm tofu found in some supermarkets and health food shops. Please use cocoa powder, not hot cocoa mix. The pudding is not pourable but very thick. You will have to scrape it out of the food processor. A blender will not work because the tofu is so thick.

Griddled Spiced Peaches

Did someone say peaches? Grab some fresh ones and start cooking. Bonus points if the juice drips down your hand like water over Niagara Falls when you slice them. Peaches are rich in potassium and vitamins A, B and C, too. At the supermarket or farmer's markets, look for peaches that give with soft pressure, have a nice aroma and no dark or mushy spots. If they aren't fully ripe, place the peaches in a brown paper bag at room temperature for a day or two to soften.

INGREDIENTS
    4 teaspoons linseed oil
    4 large ripe peaches, halved and stoned
    1½ teaspoons allspice
    1 teaspoon Truvia
    115 g/4 oz sugar-free, low-fat raspberry yoghurt

DIRECTIONS
1. Heat a large griddle pan over medium-high heat. Alternatively, prepare and heat an outdoor barbecue for direct, high-heat cooking.

2. Brush ½ teaspoon linseed oil on the cut side of each peach. Mix the mixed spice and Truvia in a small bowl and sprinkle evenly over the cut side of the peach halves.

3. Set the peaches cut side down on the griddle pan or on the barbecue grill directly over the heat. Grill until golden brown, for about 2 minutes. Turn with a wide, flat fish slice or tongs and continue grilling for 1 minute. Transfer to plates, cut side up. Put 1 tablespoon yoghurt in the centre of each peach half.

YIELD: 4 servings

TIP: Best to get freestone peaches, not cling, so that you can remove stones easily.

17 Sample Cycle 2 Menus

Here are examples of how you can create your daily menu using the preceding recipes during the Activate Cycle.

Day 1

Breakfast

☐ 1 *Dr Mike's Power Cookie*

☐ 1 fresh peach, sliced

☐ 1 cup green tea

Lunch

☐ 1 serving *Smoked Turkey and Lentil Salad*

☐ 175 g/6 oz sugar-free, fruit-flavoured yoghurt

Dinner

☐ 1 serving *Curried Poached Halibut*

☐ Steamed veggies

Snack

☐ 1 serving *Super Strawberry Smoothie*

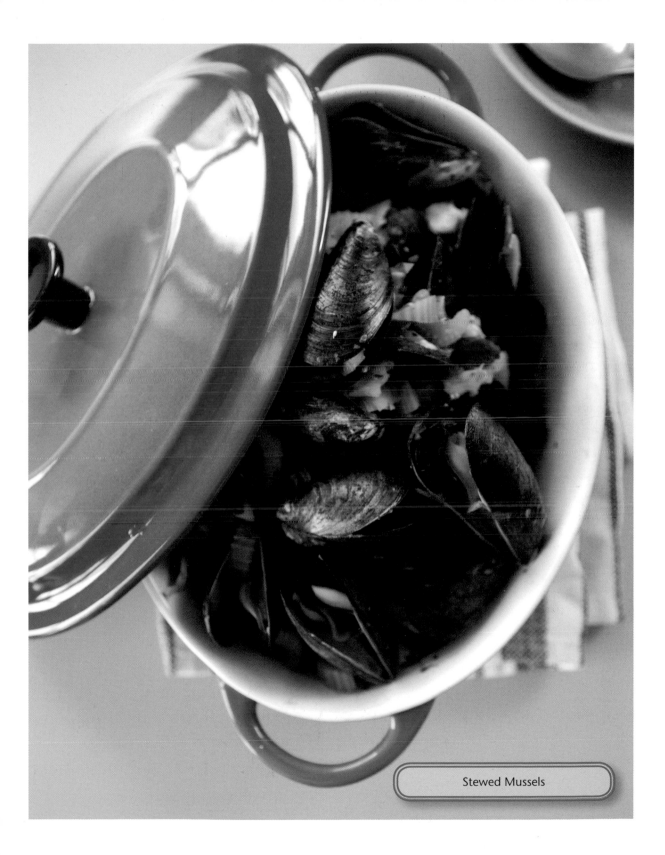

Stewed Mussels

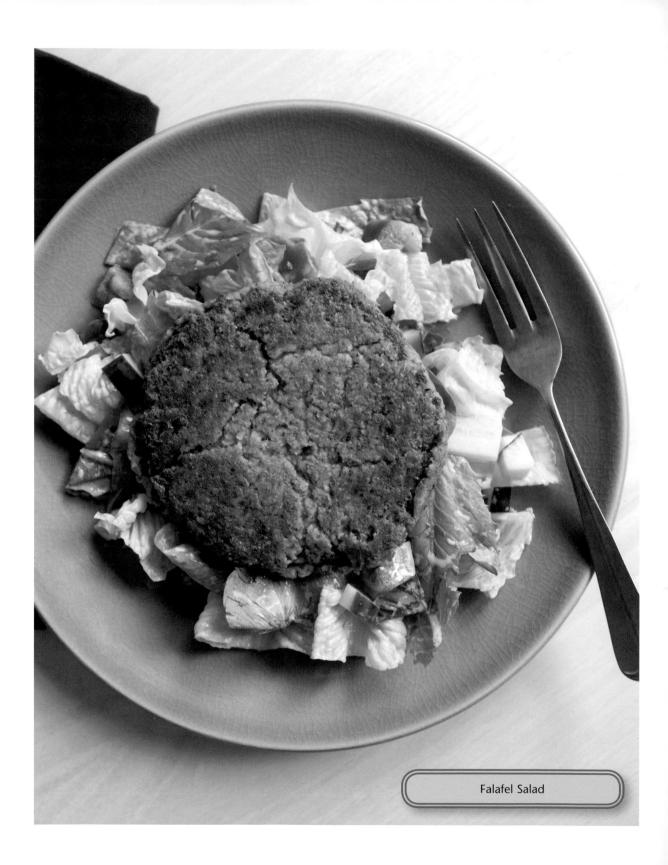

Falafel Salad

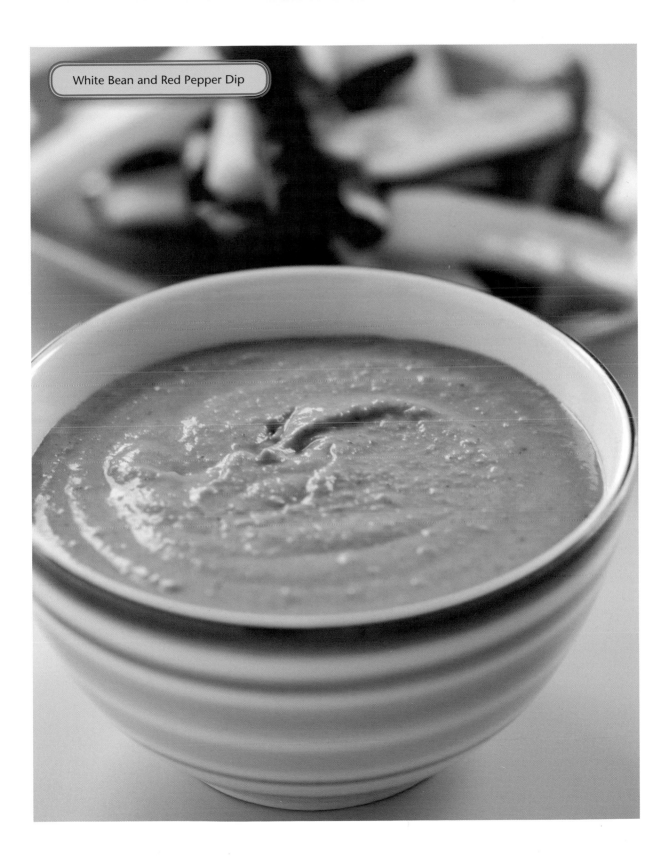

White Bean and Red Pepper Dip

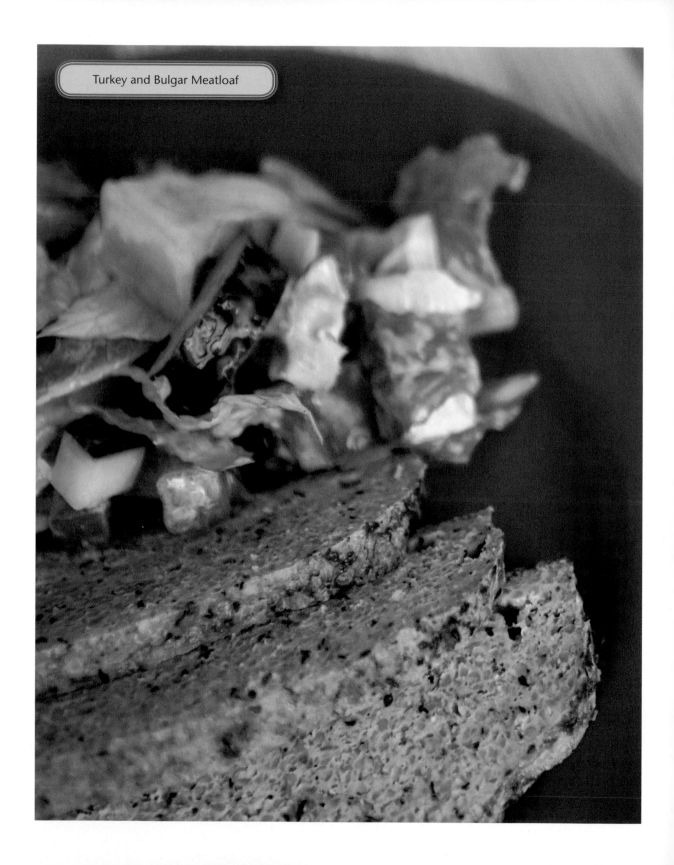

Turkey and Bulgar Meatloaf

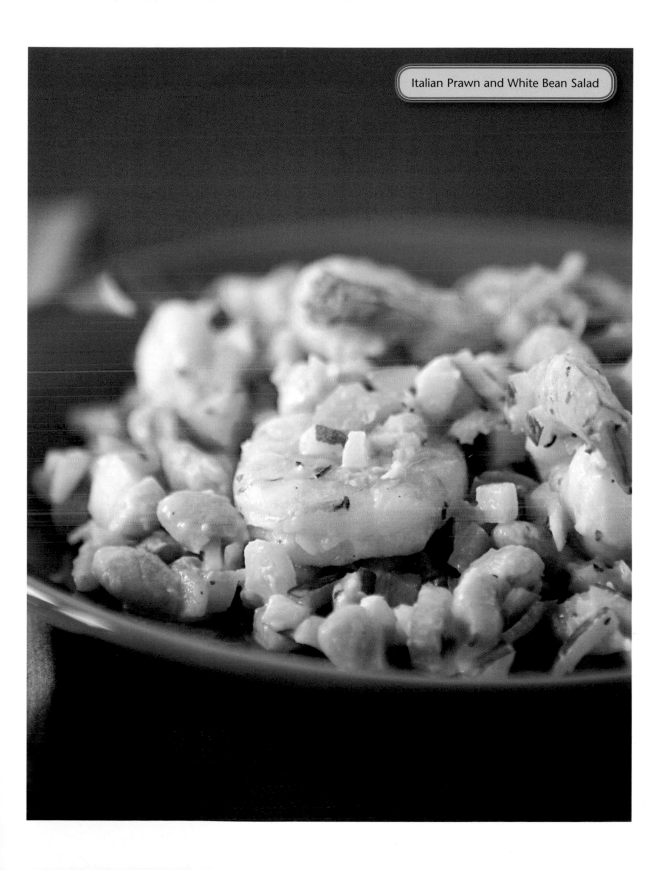

Italian Prawn and White Bean Salad

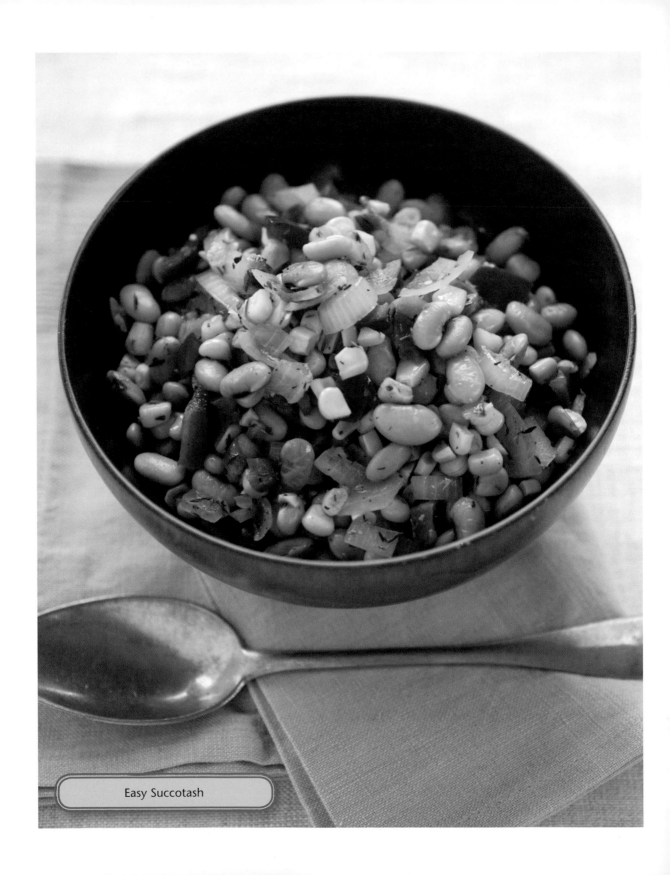

Easy Succotash

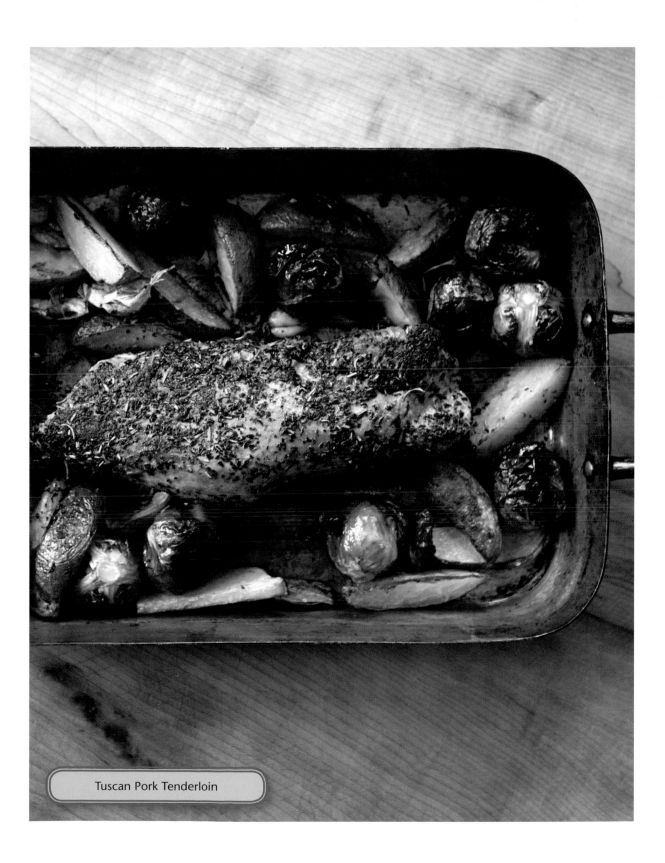

Tuscan Pork Tenderloin

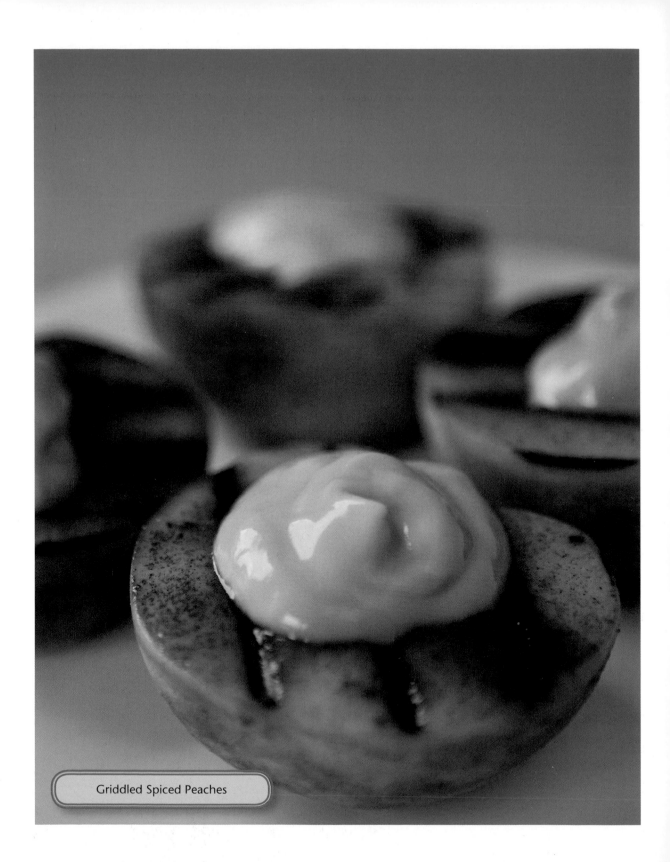

Griddled Spiced Peaches

Day 2

Breakfast

☐ 1 serving *Snappy Eggs*

☐ ½ grapefruit or other fresh fruit

☐ 1 cup green tea

Lunch

☐ 1 serving *California Tuna Salad*

☐ 1 cup green tea

Dinner

☐ 1 serving *Tandoori Chicken Breasts*

☐ 1 cup green tea

Snacks

☐ 175 g/6 oz non-fat yoghurt, sweetened with Truvia or a tablespoon of sugar-free fruit jam or other probiotic serving

☐ 1 serving of fruit from the Cycle 1 list

NOTES

Day 3

Breakfast

- ☐ 1 serving *Eggs, Salmon and Onions*
- ☐ ½ grapefruit or other fresh fruit
- ☐ 1 cup green tea

Lunch

- ☐ 1 serving *Easy Chicken Posole*
- ☐ 175 g/6 oz sugar-free, fruit-flavoured yoghurt
- ☐ 1 cup green tea

Dinner

- ☐ 1 serving *Slow-Cooker Cuban Ropa Vieja*
- ☐ 1 cup green tea

Snacks

- ☐ 125 g/4½ oz fresh raspberries or other in-season fruit with 175 g/6 oz sugar-free, fruit-flavoured yoghurt
- ☐ 1 serving *White Bean and Red Pepper Dip*

Breakfast

- ☐ 1 serving *Mushroom Spinach Frittata*
- ☐ ½ grapefruit or other fresh fruit in season
- ☐ 1 cup green tea

Lunch

- ☐ 1 large bowl of *Chicken-Vegetable Soup*
- ☐ 1 cup green tea

Dinner

- ☐ Plenty of roast turkey breast or turkey fillet, steamed carrots and steamed asparagus.
- ☐ 1 cup green tea

Snacks

- ☐ 175 g/6 oz non-fat yoghurt, sweetened with Truvia or a table-spoon of sugar-free fruit jam
- ☐ 1 serving *Kefir Smoothie*

Day 5

Breakfast

- ☐ 1 serving *Weekend Morning Polenta Bake*
- ☐ 1 fresh peach, sliced
- ☐ 1 cup green tea

Lunch

- ☐ 1 serving *Crab Tabouleh*
- ☐ 1 cup green tea

Dinner

- ☐ 1 serving *Stewed Mussels*
- ☐ 1 cup green tea

Snacks

- ☐ 150 g/5½ oz blueberries with 175 g/6 oz sugar-free, fruit-flavoured yoghurt
- ☐ 175 g/6 oz sugar-free, fruit-flavoured yoghurt or 250 ml/8 fl oz kefir

Day 6

Breakfast

☐ 175 g/6 oz natural low-fat yoghurt, mixed with 125 g/4½ oz berries, or other fruit on the Cycle 1 list sweetened with Truvia or a tablespoon of sugar-free fruit jam.

☐ 1 cup green tea

Lunch

☐ Grilled chicken breast with tossed salad drizzled with 1 table-spoon olive or linseed oil and 2 tablespoons balsamic vinegar

☐ 1 cup green tea

Dinner

☐ 1 serving *Curried Poached Halibut*

☐ 1 cup green tea

Snacks

☐ 1 serving *Griddled Spiced Peaches*

☐ Probiotic serving

NOTES

Breakfast

☐ 1 serving *Snappy Eggs*

☐ 1 orange or other fresh fruit in season

☐ 1 cup green tea

Lunch

☐ 1 serving *Fast and Easy Chilli*

☐ Large tossed salad with 1 tablespoon olive oil mixed with 2 tablespoons vinegar and seasoning

☐ 1 cup green tea

Dinner

☐ 1 serving *Turkey and Bulgar Meatloaf*

☐ 1 serving *Spicy Green Beans*

☐ 1 cup green tea

Snacks

☐ 1 serving *Kefir Smoothie*

☐ 175 g/6 oz sugar-free, fruit-flavoured yoghurt

Day 8

Breakfast

☐ 175 g/6 oz natural low-fat yoghurt, mixed with 125 g/4 ½ oz berries, or other fruit on the Cycle 1 list, sweetened with 1 sachet of Truvia or a tablespoon of sugar-free fruit jam.

☐ 1 cup green tea

Lunch

☐ 1 serving *Lemon-Pepper Salmon Salad in Tomato Cups*

☐ 1 cup green tea

Dinner

☐ Turkey burgers (made with lean turkey mince)

☐ Steamed vegetables (choose from Cycle 1 vegetables)

☐ Side salad drizzled with 1 tablespoon olive or linseed oil, mixed with 2 tablespoons balsamic vinegar and seasonings

☐ 1 cup green tea

Snack

☐ 1 serving *Berry Frozen Yoghurt*

Day 9

Breakfast

- ☐ 115 g/4 oz natural cottage cheese
- ☐ 1 medium pear, sliced
- ☐ 1 cup green tea

Lunch

- ☐ Grilled chicken breast
- ☐ 1 serving *Butternut Squash Polenta*
- ☐ 1 cup green tea

Dinner

- ☐ Grilled salmon
- ☐ Steamed broccoli
- ☐ 1 serving *Mexican Chocolate Pudding*
- ☐ 1 cup green tea

Snacks

- ☐ 1 medium apple
- ☐ 175 g/6 oz sugar-free, fruit-flavoured yoghurt

Day 10

Breakfast

☐ 1 serving *Spanish Omelette*

☐ ½ grapefruit or 1 medium orange

☐ 1 cup green tea

Lunch

☐ 1 serving *Creamy Smoked Salmon Rolls*

☐ 1 cup green tea

Dinner

☐ Plenty of roast turkey breast or turkey fillet, steamed carrots and steamed asparagus

☐ 1 cup green tea

Snacks

☐ 1 piece fresh fruit

☐ 175 g/6 oz non-fat yoghurt

Day 11

Breakfast

- ☐ 1 serving *Kefir Smoothie*
- ☐ 1 cup green tea

Lunch

- ☐ Plenty of grilled beefburger
- ☐ 1 serving *Microwave Mashed Potatoes*

Dinner

- ☐ 1 serving *Tuscan Pork Tenderloin*
- ☐ Steamed asparagus
- ☐ Large tossed salad with 1 tablespoon olive oil mixed with 2 tablespoons vinegar and seasoning

Snacks

- ☐ 1 medium orange
- ☐ 175 g/6 oz sugar-free, fruit-flavoured yoghurt

Day 12

Breakfast

- ☐ 1 serving *Yoghurt Fruitshake*
- ☐ 1 cup green tea

Lunch

- ☐ 1 serving *Super Salad*
- ☐ 1 cup green tea

Dinner

- ☐ Steamed plaice or sole with lemon pepper
- ☐ Steamed broccoli
- ☐ 1 cup green tea

Snacks

- ☐ 1 medium apple, or other fruit in season
- ☐ 1 serving *Berry Frozen Yoghurt*

NOTES

Breakfast

- ☐ 1 *Dr Mike's Power Cookie*
- ☐ 1 medium peach, sliced
- ☐ 1 cup green tea

Lunch

- ☐ Fruit salad: 115 g/4 oz natural cottage cheese with 85 g/3 oz diced strawberries and 85 g/3 oz diced peach served on a generous bed of lettuce
- ☐ 1 cup green tea

Dinner

- ☐ 1 serving *Roast Prawns and Broccoli*
- ☐ 1 cup green tea

Snacks

- ☐ 1 serving *Yoghurt Fruitshake*
- ☐ 1 serving *Berry Frozen Yoghurt*

Day 14

Breakfast

☐ 1 serving *Peach Melba Smoothie*

☐ 1 cup green tea

Lunch

☐ 1 serving *Super Salad*

☐ 1 cup green tea

Dinner

☐ 1 serving *Blackened Mahi-Mahi* with liberal amounts of any Cycle 1 vegetables, steamed or raw

☐ 1 cup green tea

Snacks

☐ 175 g/6 oz sugar-free, fruit-flavoured yoghurt, or 225 g/8 oz natural low-fat yoghurt, sweetened with Truvia or a tablespoon of sugar-free fruit jam

☐ 1 serving of fruit

NOTES

Day 15

Breakfast

- ☐ 115 g/4 oz cooked porridge
- ☐ 175 g/6 oz sugar-free, fruit-flavoured yoghurt
- ☐ 1 cup green tea

Lunch

- ☐ 1 serving *Cantonese Stir-fried Prawns*
- ☐ 1 cup green tea

Dinner

- ☐ 1 serving *Turkey and Bulgar Meatloaf*
- ☐ 1 cup green tea

Snacks

- ☐ 1 medium apple or pear
- ☐ 2nd probiotic serving

Day 16

Breakfast

- ☐ 2 scrambled egg whites
- ☐ ½ grapefruit or other fresh fruit in season
- ☐ 1 cup green tea

Lunch

- ☐ 1 large bowl of *Chicken-Vegetable Soup*
- ☐ 1 cup green tea

Dinner

- ☐ 1 serving *Stir-Fried Chicken and Cucumbers*
- ☐ 1 cup green tea

Snacks

- ☐ 125 g/4½ oz fresh berries
- ☐ 175 g/6 oz non-fat yoghurt, sweetened with Truvia or a tablespoon of sugar-free fruit jam

Day 17

Breakfast

☐ 1 serving *Eggs, Salmon and Onions*

☐ 125 g/4½ oz fresh berries

☐ 1 cup green tea

Lunch

☐ 1 serving *Italian Prawn and White Bean Salad*

☐ 1 cup green tea

Dinner

☐ 1 serving *Bavarian Chicken Breasts*

☐ 1 cup green tea

Snacks

☐ 1 medium orange or nectarine

☐ 2nd probiotic serving

RECIPES

Cycle 3 – Achieve

GOAL: To develop good eating habits through the reintroduction of additional foods and move you closer to your goal weight.

Better Migas

I love migas (MEE-gahs), a spicy Mexican concoction of tortillas scrambled with eggs, peppers and beans, topped with salsa. On a good morning, I prefer my migas with a shot of hot sauce. This recipe has all the robust flavour of traditional migas without the fat and calories. It's high in fibre, too, thanks to the addition of pinto beans. Eggs, of course, are the ultimate protein: they digest easily, help prevent fat deposits and are good for memory and concentration.

INGREDIENTS

400 g/14 oz canned pinto beans, drained and rinsed

1 canned chipotle chilli in adobo sauce, stem removed

2 tablespoons lime juice

1 tablespoon chilli powder

½ teaspoon garlic powder

½ teaspoon salt

2 x 25-cm/10-inch wholemeal tortillas

Non-stick cooking spray

2 medium eggs

60 g/2¼ oz prepared salsa

2 tablespoons grated low-fat Cheddar cheese

DIRECTIONS

1. Place the pinto beans, chipotle, lime juice, 2 tablespoons water, chilli powder, garlic powder and salt in a large processor. Cover and process until fairly smooth, like refried beans, scraping down the inside of the bowl once or twice. Set aside.

2. Set a large non-stick frying pan over a medium heat for 1 minute. Add the tortillas one at a time and cook, turning once, until warmed and a little browned, for about 1 minute. Transfer to two plates. Spread each of the tortillas with 4 tablespoons of the bean mixture. Wipe out the pan.

(continued on next page)

Better Migas (*cont.*)

3. Spray the non-stick frying pan with non-stick cooking spray and set over the heat for 1 minute. Crack the eggs into the pan. Cook until the whites are set but the yolks are soft, for about 3 minutes, flipping after 2 minutes. (Alternatively, cook for about 2½ minutes without flipping; for harder cooked yolks, cook 1 minute longer after flipping.) Use a wide palette knife to set a fried egg on each tortilla. Top each with 2 tablespoons salsa and 1 tablespoon grated cheese.

YIELD: 2 servings

> **TIPS:** Using this recipe, you've essentially made mock refried beans, much lower in fat but just as tasty. It'll make more than you need, which is a good thing, because the leftovers can be served as a dip or as a side dish. Store it, covered, in the fridge. It can be heated in the microwave for a minute or two. Make sure you use 1 canned chipotle in adobo sauce, not 1 can of chipotles. Find them in most supermarkets near the canned refried beans and other Mexican foods.

Slow-cooker Brown Rice Congee

Doctors don't have lots of time to read, but when we do, we read medical journals, which sounds kind of boring. The last journal I read was the Journal of Chinese Medicine, *in which I learnt about* congee, *a creamy rice soup that is a traditional breakfast food in China. It sounded perfect for the 17 Day Diet, so I include my brown-rice version here. The article, by the way, linked eating congee to living longer. I suppose that means you can enjoy your fit, trim body longer by adding this tasty, light and healthy breakfast food to your menu.*

INGREDIENTS

- 1.9 litres/3½ pints vegetable stock
- 200 g/7 oz medium-grain brown rice, such as brown Arborio rice
- 1 tablespoon peeled, finely chopped, fresh root ginger or 1 tablespoon ready-prepared finely chopped root ginger

Suggested garnishes

Thinly sliced spring onions

Chopped, skinless boneless chicken breast

Chopped, cooked prawns

Diced firm tofu

Dry roasted salted peanuts

Asian hot sauce, such as sambal olek or sriracha

DIRECTIONS

1. Stir the stock, rice and ginger in a 5- to 6-litre/8½- to 10-pint slow cooker. Cover and cook on low until creamy and porridge-like, for about 10 hours.

2. To serve, ladle 250-ml/8-fl-oz servings into bowls. Sprinkle with small amounts of one or more garnishes. Or skip the toppings altogether and enjoy the congee as a hot, savoury, breakfast cereal on its own.

YIELD: 8 servings

(continued on next page)

Slow-cooker Brown Rice Congee (*cont.*)

TIP: Leftovers can be refrigerated, then reheated in a microwave or a small saucepan the next day. If too stiff after refrigerating, loosen the dish with a little extra stock or water before reheating. This is a great recipe for weekend company or a holiday breakfast alternative.

Breakfast Pizza Bagels

Leftover pizza for breakfast? Admit it: you've eaten it. Maybe not the best choice but it does hit the spot occasionally, especially when there's nothing else in the fridge. Not to worry. This nutritious, filling recipe now makes it legitimate to eat pizza for breakfast.

INGREDIENTS

- 1 wholegrain bagel, split in half
- 115 g/4 oz reduced-fat Emmenthal cheese, thinly sliced
- 2 teaspoons finely chopped chives or the green part of a spring onion
- 4 thin tomato slices
- ½ teaspoon salt

DIRECTIONS

1. Position a shelf 10 to 15 cm/4 to 6 inches from the grill and pre-heat the grill. Set the bagel halves cut side up on a baking tray. Grill until brown and toasty, for about 2 minutes.

2. Remove the baking tray from the oven and leave the grill on. Top each bagel half with half the sliced cheese, 1 teaspoon finely chopped chives, 2 tomato slices and ¼ teaspoon salt. Grill until the tomatoes are bubbling and the cheese has melted, for about 2 minutes.

YIELD: 2 servings

> **TIPS:** You don't want seeds or other toppings on the bagel because they can burn in the intense grill heat. Use a large slicing tomato for the best slices. Don't like chives? Try some thyme leaves or finely chopped oregano leaves.

Banana Chocolate Smoothie

If you're craving something chocolatey, why not set your sights on something truly worth coveting? I'm talking about a delicious, creamy chocolate smoothie to kick-start your day. With the addition of a banana and silken tofu, this is one smoothie that tastes decadent, but has huge health pay-offs: lots of fibre, low in fat and if you opt for soya milk, it's dairy-, gluten- and lactose-free.

INGREDIENTS

1 small banana, peeled and cut into 2.5-cm/1-inch pieces

125 g/4½ oz soft silken tofu

125 ml/4 fl oz soya milk or skimmed milk

3 tablespoons sugar-free chocolate-flavored syrup

1 teaspoon Truvia

DIRECTIONS

Place all the ingredients in a blender. Cover and blend until smooth, turning off the machine and scraping down the inside of the container at least once.

YIELD: 1 serving (can be doubled)

> **TIPS:** Want it colder? Add an ice cube. Want more texture? Add 1 tablespoon toasted wheat germ.

White Bean and Oat Burgers

There are plenty of meat substitutes like vegetarian and vegan burgers in the marketplace, and for the most part, they taste pretty good. Or least I thought so, until I tasted these. Delicious. You won't be asking "Where's the beef?" you'll be asking, "Who needs the beef?"

INGREDIENTS

- 400 g/14 oz canned cannellini beans, drained and rinsed
- 50 g/1¾ oz porridge oats (do not use quick-cooking or steel-cut oats)
- 55 g/2 oz (about 24) whole roasted almonds (do not use salted almonds)
- 1 medium egg
- 1 tablespoon finely chopped sage leaves or 1½ teaspoons dried sage
- 1 teaspoon salt
- ½ teaspoon ground black pepper
- ¼ teaspoon garlic powder
- ¼ teaspoon onion powder
- 1 tablespoon olive oil
- 4 wholemeal pitta pockets
- Chopped iceberg lettuce
- 125 ml/4 fl oz low-fat, sugar-free bottled ranch dressing

DIRECTIONS

1. Place the beans, oats, almonds, egg, sage, salt, pepper, garlic powder and onion powder in a food processor fitted with the chopping blade. Cover and process until pasty, scraping down the inside of the bowl once or twice.

2. Scrape down and remove the chopping blade. Use wet hands to scoop up and pat the mixture into four equal burgers, each about 13 cm/5 inches in diameter.

3. Heat the oil in a large non-stick frying pan over a medium heat. Slip the burgers into the frying pan and cook until browned and firm, for about 8 minutes, turning once. Serve the burgers in the

(continued on next page)

White Bean and Oat Burgers (*cont.*)

pitta pockets, each stuffed with chopped lettuce and drizzled with 2 tablespoons ranch dressing.

YIELD: 4 servings

TIP: The burgers can be cooked and kept covered in the fridge. To recrisp them, heat in a dry frying pan over a medium heat, for about 4 minutes, turning once, or place them on a baking sheet and bake for about 10 minutes in a preheated oven at Gas Mark 4/180°C/fan oven 160°C.

Open-faced Reuben

Every so often I get a real craving for a Reuben sandwich. However, the traditional American sandwich includes high-fat Russian or Thousand Island dressing, corned beef and Swiss cheese, and it is fried in butter. We slimmed down the Reuben by using turkey pastrami, low-fat Russian dressing and low-fat Emmenthal cheese. Instead of frying the sandwich in butter, you carefully grill it. And, let me tell you, this retooled Reuben is magnificent.

INGREDIENTS
2 slices pumpernickel bread or rye bread

2 tablespoons low-fat prepared Russian dressing

55 g/2 oz turkey pastrami, thinly sliced

4 thin tomato slices

150 g/5½ oz bottled sauerkraut, drained and rinsed

85 g/3 oz low-fat Emmenthal cheese, thinly sliced

DIRECTIONS
1. Position the oven shelf 10 to 15 cm/4 to 6 inches from the grill. Lay the bread slices on a baking tray and toast until crunchy, for about 3 minutes, turning once. Remove from the oven and leave the grill on.

2. Spread each slice with 1 tablespoon Russian dressing. Top with half the turkey pastrami, 2 tomato slices, half the sauerkraut and half the cheese. Grill until the cheese has melted and is beginning to brown, for about 3 minutes.

YIELD: 2 servings (can be doubled)

> **TIPS:** Turkey pastrami is available at some supermarkets and online. Drain the sauerkraut well, even squeezing it a bit by handfuls over the sink. You don't want excess moisture to make the bread soggy.

Brie and Mango Quesadilla

Gourmet meets Tex-Mex, and it's a marriage made in culinary heaven. And so quick to make. In less than 10 minutes, you've got a meal. Now, that's my kind of lunch.

INGREDIENTS

2 x 25-cm/10-inch wholemeal tortillas
115 g/4 oz Brie, rind removed
1 large mango, peeled, stoned and thinly sliced
1 roasted red pepper, cut in half
Non-stick cooking spray

DIRECTIONS

1. Lay one tortilla on a work surface. Spread half the cheese over half the tortilla. Lay half the mango and half the roasted red pepper over the cheese. Fold the tortilla to make a semicircle. Repeat with the other tortilla.

2. Spray a large non-stick frying pan with non-stick cooking spray. Set over a medium heat for 1 minute. Add the quesadillas and cook until the tortilla is lightly browned and the cheese has melted, for about 4 minutes, turning once.

YIELD: 2 servings (can be doubled)

> **TIP:** You can find ready-sliced mango in the produce section of most supermarkets. One traditional way to make quesadillas is to weigh them down in the frying pan, making them flatter and crisper. Use a heavy pot lid or even a large saucepan, pressing a bit as it first sits on top of them. Or put a lightweight lid on them and top with a 400-g/14-oz can of beans.

Crab Gazpacho

Gazpacho is the king of cold soups. It brings together a veritable garden of healthy veggies all in one bowl. Ours is souped up with crabmeat for an extra punch of protein, resulting in a complete meal that's healthy, simple and easy to make.

INGREDIENTS

2 large tomatoes, finely chopped, all juice reserved
1 medium green pepper, deseeded and finely chopped
1 large carrot, peeled and coarsely grated
2 celery sticks, finely chopped
½ large cucumber, peeled, deseeded and finely chopped
30 g/1 oz red onion, finally chopped
2 tablespoons Worcestershire sauce
1 tablespoon lemon juice
Several dashes Tabasco sauce
135 g/4¾ oz canned crabmeat

DIRECTIONS

Stir the tomatoes, green pepper, carrot, celery, cucumber, red onion, Worcestershire sauce, lemon juice and Tabasco sauce in a medium bowl. Divide between 2 serving bowls and top each with half the crabmeat.

YIELD: 2 servings (can be doubled)

TIPS: The trick here is to finely chop the vegetables so they're all about the same size, so that you can have different flavours and textures in every spoonful.

The soup keeps well in the fridge, covered, for up to 3 days. Can be served cold. If taking for lunch, put the crabmeat in a separate container, then add when you are ready to eat.

Spinach Mushroom Salad
with Warm Bacon Dressing

Most versions of this popular salad are rather weighty due to the amount of bacon used. This recipe relies on a lower-fat alternative: turkey bacon. The addition of feta cheese and mushrooms adds to this salad's tastiness.

INGREDIENTS

115 g/4 oz baby spinach leaves

115 g/4 oz white button or chestnut mushrooms, thinly sliced

2 teaspoons olive oil

4 rashers turkey bacon, chopped

1 tablespoon finely chopped shallot

1 tablespoon apple-cider vinegar

1 teaspoon Dijon mustard

55 g/2 oz feta cheese

½ teaspoon ground black pepper

DIRECTIONS

1. Toss the spinach and mushrooms in a large bowl. Set aside.

2. Heat the oil in a non-stick frying pan over a medium heat. Add the bacon and cook, stirring often, until crisp, for about 3 minutes. Add the shallots and stir over the heat for 30 seconds to soften them. Stir in the vinegar and mustard. Pour the warm dressing over the spinach and mushrooms and toss well.

3. Divide the salad between 2 plates. Top each with half the feta and the black pepper.

YIELD: 2 servings (can be doubled)

TIP: The hot dressing should wilt the spinach leaves a bit.

Tex-Mex Millet Salad

Here's one of the healthiest and highest fibre salads you'll ever make. It spotlights two unusual ingredients: nutty-tasting millet, *a nutritious gluten-free grain that's a staple cereal in Africa, Asia and India; and* jicama *(pronounced hee-ka-ma), a low-calorie root vegetable available at West Indian grocery shops with an apple-like texture. Jicama contains a group of fibres known as* fructans, *specifically* inulin, *which helps promote bone and digestive health. Added to the salad are other high-fibre goodies: pinto beans, sweetcorn, almonds and plums.*

INGREDIENTS

- 50 g/2 oz millet (do not use millet grits)
- 250 g/9 oz canned pinto beans, drained and rinsed
- 115 g/4 oz canned chopped roasted green chillies, hot or mild
- 1 small jicama, peeled and chopped
- 1 large ripe, red plum, stoned and chopped
- 80 g/2¾ oz frozen sweetcorn niblets, thawed
- 25 g/1 oz flaked almonds
- 2 tablespoons lime juice
- 2 teaspoons chilli powder
- 1 teaspoon olive oil or walnut oil (optional)

DIRECTIONS

1. Bring 300 ml/10 fl oz water to the boil over a high heat. Stir in the millet. Cover, reduce the heat to low and simmer until the water has been absorbed and the millet is tender, for about 25 minutes.

2. Scrape the millet into a large bowl. Stir in the beans, chillies, jicama, plum, sweetcorn, almonds, lime juice, chilli powder and oil, if using.

YIELD: 2 servings (can be doubled)

> **TIP:** Once the millet is cooked, don't let it sit around or it'll start to firm up. Tip it into the bowl and stir in the remaining ingredients to keep the grains separate and soft. Store in a sealed container in the fridge for up to 3 days.

Prawn Soba Noodle Salad

Pasta salad has lots of loyal fans, and this recipe will create many more. It's made with soba, a Japanese noodle usually made from buckwheat and wheat flour. Soba noodles are a health food: thanks to the buckwheat, they contain rutin, *a natural plant compound believed to help reduce blood pressure and strengthen blood vessels. Rutin may even have anticancer properties. The addition of prawns to this flavourful pasta salad adds low-fat protein to the mix. So use your noodle, your soba noodles, that is, and enjoy an Oriental rendition of a pasta salad.*

INGREDIENTS

> 2 tablespoons unseasoned rice vinegar
> 1 tablespoon light soy sauce
> 2 teaspoons toasted sesame oil
> 1 teaspoon peeled, finely chopped fresh root ginger
> 115 g/4 oz cooked soba noodles
> 175 g/6 oz cooked prawns, chopped
> 1 large carrot, coarsely grated
> 1 small red pepper, deseeded, and thinly sliced
> 2 medium spring onions, thinly sliced
> 2 tablespoons finely chopped fresh coriander leaves

DIRECTIONS

1. Whisk the vinegar, soy sauce, sesame oil, and ginger in a large bowl.

2. Add the noodles, prawns, carrot, red pepper, spring onions and fresh coriander. Toss well.

YIELD: 2 servings (can be doubled)

TIPS: Cook 55 g/2 oz fresh soba noodles in a big pot of boiling water to get 115 g/4 oz cooked soba noodles.

Use toasted sesame oil for the most flavour; once opened, store it in the fridge to preserve its freshness. It may solidify somewhat but will regain its liquidity after sitting at room temperature for 10 minutes.

If you're taking this to work, pack the dressing separately, so the vegetables stay fresh and crisp.

Easy Cioppino

There's nothing better than a steaming cup of authentic cioppino Italian–American (pronounced cha-pe-no), a wonderful fish stew with a rich, spicy tomato base loaded with herbs. I love it. I could bathe in it, and would happily agree to an IV of it, if that's what the doctor ordered, and I'm the doctor. This recipe, usually served in waterside restaurants, is so authentic that I can hear the seagulls in the San Diego Bay. Soup's on!

INGREDIENTS

800 g/1 lb 12 oz canned chopped tomatoes

250 ml/8 fl oz vegetable stock

1 medium white onion, chopped

1 medium fennel bulb, trimmed and chopped

1 medium green pepper, deseeded, and chopped

2 celery sticks, chopped

1 medium garlic clove, finely chopped, or 1 teaspoon ready-prepared finely chopped garlic

2 teaspoons dried basil

2 teaspoons dried oregano

½ teaspoon dried chilli flakes

225 g/8 oz halibut, cut into 2.5-cm/1-inch cubes

450 g/1 lb mussels, cleaned and debearded

DIRECTIONS

1. Bring the tomatoes, stock, onion, fennel, green pepper, celery, garlic, basil, oregano and chilli flakes to a simmer in a large saucepan set over a high heat. Cover, reduce the heat to very low and simmer for 30 minutes.

2. Add the halibut and mussels. Cover and continue simmering until the mussels open, for about 10 minutes. Discard any mussels that do not open.

YIELD: 4 servings

TIP: To save time, use 125 g/4½ oz frozen chopped onion and 150 g/5½ frozen pepper strips instead of the fresh vegetables. Thaw the frozen vegetables before using. For information on cleaning and debearding mussels, see page 77.

Roasted Trout Almandine

I've eaten lots of Trout Almandine at restaurants, and this version rivals anything I've tasted. It's so moist and flavourful, you'd think the fish had been swimming in a river of butter. No butter is used here, however, so we keep the fat and calories well below stratospheric range.

INGREDIENTS

Non-stick cooking spray
2 small whole trout, boned and cleaned
1 medium lemon, cut into 6 paper-thin slices and 2 wedges
4 fresh thyme sprigs
40 g/1½ oz flaked almonds
½ teaspoon salt
½ teaspoon black pepper

DIRECTIONS

1. Position a shelf in the centre of the oven and preheat to Gas Mark 6/200°C/fan oven 180°C.

2. Spray a roasting tin or the grill pan with non-stick cooking spray. Lay the trout in the tin and layer the lemon slices and thyme in the body cavity of each of the trout. Place 1 tablespoon flaked almonds in each trout as well. Close the fish and sprinkle the remaining almonds over the top. Season with salt and pepper.

3. Bake until the flesh flakes when tested with a fork, for 12 to 15 minutes. Remove from the oven and squeeze the lemon wedges over the trout and almonds. Cut each trout in half across to serve.

YIELD: 4 servings

> **TIPS:** Make sure you get boned, cleaned trout. Even so, if you're sharing a trout with a child, check for bones, particularly along the dorsal fin along the spine at the top. If you're squeamish, ask the fishmonger to remove the heads for you.

Red Snapper Veracruz

Red snapper is a white firm-fleshed fish that benefits from a spicy treatment, which this wonderfully rendered dish has. Red Snapper Veracruz style is a classic Mexican dish in which the fish is baked in a zippy sauce made with tomatoes, peppers and capers. Enjoy!

INGREDIENTS

- 800 g/1 lb 12 oz canned chopped tomatoes
- 1 medium red pepper, deseeded and chopped
- 1 medium green pepper, deseeded and chopped
- 10 bottled, pickled jalapeño slices, drained and chopped, or to taste
- 15 g/½ oz fresh parsley leaves, chopped
- 1 tablespoon fresh thyme leaves or 2 teaspoons dried thyme
- 1 teaspoon drained and rinsed capers, chopped
- ½ teaspoon salt
- 4 skinless red snapper fillets, about 115 g/4 oz each

DIRECTIONS

1. Bring the tomatoes, peppers, jalapeño, parsley, thyme, capers and salt to a simmer in a large saucepan set over a medium-high heat. Cover, reduce the heat to low and simmer slowly for 20 minutes.

2. Slip the fish fillets into the tomato mixture. Cover and cook until the fish flakes when tested with a fork, for about 10 minutes. Ladle the soup and fish into bowls to serve.

YIELD: 4 servings

> **TIP:** To save time, use 300 g/10 oz frozen pepper strips, thawed, instead of the red and green peppers. You'll have strips, not chopped pepper, but that won't matter much, except for the look of the dish.

Grilled Miso-glazed Salmon

Using a glaze on this favourite fish is a fast way to add flavour without having to marinate the salmon. This sweet-and-sour glaze gets its flavour from soy sauce, no-sugar-added apricot jam or all-fruit spread, and miso paste. Miso is a mixture of cooked soya beans, salt and a steamed grain such as rice, wheat or barley that has been injected with a mould culture to stimulate fermentation. Miso's flavour has been described in hundreds of ways, including rich, earthy, tangy, beany, nutty, buttery, mushroomy, meaty and salty.

INGREDIENTS

75 g/2½ oz white miso paste

3 tablespoons unseasoned rice vinegar

3 tablespoons light soy sauce

2 tablespoons sugar-free apricot jam or all-fruit spread

1 tablespoon peeled, finely chopped, fresh root ginger or ready-prepared, finely chopped root ginger

4 skinless salmon fillets, about 115 g/4 oz each

DIRECTIONS

1. Stir the miso paste, rice vinegar, soy sauce, apricot jam, and ginger in a large bowl.

2. Spread the miso mixture on both sides of each fillet and place on a baking tray.

3. Position the shelf 10 to 15 cm/4 to 6 inches from the grill and preheat the grill.

4. Set the tray on the shelf and grill for 4 minutes. Use a large fish slice to turn the fillets and continue grilling until the salmon flakes when tested with a fork, for about a further 4 more minutes.

YIELD: 4 servings

> **TIP:** There are several kinds of miso; make sure you use the milder white.

Prawn Vindaloo

Vindaloo is a spicy curry. Grapes counterbalance all the spices, with a flavour combo that will enliven your palate.

INGREDIENTS

1 teaspoon salt

½ teaspoon mustard powder

½ teaspoon ground coriander

½ teaspoon ground cumin

½ teaspoon ground ginger

½ teaspoon turmeric

¼ to ½ teaspoon cayenne

¼ teaspoon ground cinnamon

⅛ teaspoon ground cloves

1½ tablespoons red wine vinegar

Non-stick cooking spray

1 large white onion, chopped

3 tablespoons peeled, finely chopped, fresh root ginger or ready prepared, finely chopped root ginger

3 medium garlic cloves, finely chopped, or 1 tablespoon ready prepared finely chopped garlic

300 ml/10 fl oz vegetable stock

16 seedless white grapes, halved

450 g/1 lb (about 30) peeled, de-veined medium prawns

DIRECTIONS

1. Mix the salt, mustard, coriander, cumin, ginger, turmeric, cayenne, cinnamon and cloves in a small bowl. Stir in the vinegar to make a paste. Set aside.

2. Spray a large saucepan with non-stick cooking spray and set over a medium heat for 1 minute. Add the onion and cook, stirring often, until softened, for about 4 minutes.

3. Add the ginger and garlic and cook for 20 seconds. Add the spice paste and cook for 30 seconds, until aromatic. Stir in the stock and

(continued on next page)

Prawn Vindaloo (*cont.*)

grapes. Reduce the heat to medium-low and simmer, uncovered, for 10 minutes.

4. Add the prawns, raise the heat to medium-high and cook for 4 minutes, until the prawns are pink and firm.

YIELD: 4 servings

> **TIPS:** Vindaloo is usually served with rice because the starch cuts the heat. You can use brown rice here. However, it's just as good on a bed of cucumber noodles. Simply use a vegetable peeler to create long, thin noodles from peeled cucumbers, stopping when you get to the seedy core.
>
> To save a little time, omit the first 9 ingredients; use 1 tablespoon Madras curry powder, or another hot curry powder, and mix the red wine vinegar into it. (Vindaloo curry powder is often unbalanced in flavour.) You may need to add salt to taste at the end of the recipe if the curry powder you use doesn't include salt.

Arroz con Poussins

Ask a Latin-American like me where to find a good arroz con pollo recipe and the answer is usually: "At my mum's." Arroz con pollo (rice with chicken) is a hearty, satisfying, inexpensive dish that's a meal in itself. It's usually made in one pan or a flameproof ovenproof dish on the hob, with chicken stock and spices added to the chicken's juices. Saffron turns the rice golden, and peas top the dish. It's easy and appealing, perfect for a healthy family dinner or for company. Here we make it with nutrient-packed brown rice and poussins, a flavourful, tender variation on a classic Latino dish.

INGREDIENTS

1 tablespoon olive oil

2 x 450 g/1 lb poussins, skinned and halved lengthways

1 small white onion, chopped

1 medium green pepper, deseeded, and chopped

2 medium garlic cloves, finely chopped, or 2 teaspoons ready-prepared finely chopped garlic

400 g/14 oz canned chopped tomatoes

140 g/5 oz brown basmati rice

2 teaspoons dried oregano

½ teaspoon ground allspice

½ teaspoon salt

½ teaspoon ground black pepper

¼ teaspoon saffron, optional

500 ml/16 fl oz fat-free, low-sodium chicken stock

150 g/5½ oz frozen green peas

DIRECTIONS

1. Heat the oil in a large wide pan. Put the poussins in the pan and brown on both sides for about 10 minutes, turning once. Transfer the poussins to a chopping board or a bowl.

2. Add the onion, green pepper and garlic to the pot and cook, stirring often, until softened, for about 4 minutes. Pour in the

(continued on next page)

Arroz con Poussins (*cont.*)

chopped tomatoes and all their juices and stir in the rice, oregano, mixed spice, salt, pepper and saffron, if using. Bring to a simmer, then stir over the heat until the tomatoes begin to break down, for about 2 minutes.

3. Pour in the stock, nestle the poussins into the pan and sprinkle the peas over the top. Cover, reduce the heat to low and simmer until the rice is tender and the liquid is almost all absorbed, for about 50 minutes. Set aside for 10 minutes to allow the flavours to infuse.

YIELD: 4 servings

TIPS: Ask a butcher to skin and halve the poussins for you or buy spatchcocked birds. Because of liquid content and cooking times, you can't use white rice with this dish. It has to be made with brown. You can use brown Thai fragrant rice for a more aromatic dish. The secret to keeping the poussins from sticking is to leave them to brown and keep going, undisturbed. They'll brown, caramelise and then those natural sugars will release from the pot and you can pop the birds off the base of the pot. Moving and nudging them starts the process all over, with new sugars exposed, and more sticking.

Crab Cakes

It's not easy to reduce crab cakes into something you can enjoy whilst losing weight, but this recipe succeeds. With the addition of low-fat mayonnaise, they're moist and delicious with a perfect spicy tang. Using wholemeal breadcrumbs spikes up the nutrition.

INGREDIENTS

Non-stick cooking spray

½ small white onion, finely chopped

1 celery stick, finely chopped

225 g/8 oz crabmeat

2 tablespoons low-fat mayonnaise

2 tablespoons wholemeal breadcrumbs

1 tablespoon Dijon mustard

1 teaspoon Cajun seasoning blend

60 ml/2 fl oz sugar-free cocktail sauce or calorie-free seafood sauce

DIRECTIONS

1. Spray a large frying pan, preferably non-stick, with non-stick cooking spray. Set over a medium heat, then add the onion and celery. Cook, stirring often, until the onion softens, for about 3 minutes. Transfer the vegetables to a large bowl and leave to cool for 5 minutes. Set the pan aside.

2. Add the crabmeat, mayonnaise, breadcrumbs, mustard and spice blend to the bowl. Stir gently to create a uniform mixture. Divide into four even cakes, about 7.5-cm/¾-inch thick, patting them between your palms to make sure they cohere.

3. Spray the pan again with non-stick cooking spray and set over a medium heat for 1 minute. Slip the crab cakes into the pan and cook until brown and crunchy, for about 8 minutes, turning once. Serve each cake with 1 tablespoon cocktail sauce.

YIELD: 4 servings

(continued on next page)

Crab Cakes (*cont.*)

TIPS: The trick here is to chop the celery as finely as possible so there are no chunks in the final cakes. Ready-chopped celery from the produce section won't work unless you chop the bits more finely at home.

Also, don't use canned crabmeat, found next to the canned tuna. Look for the containers at the fish counter in some supermarkets, or from a fishmonger. No need to buy anything fancy since you're mixing it with other ingredients.

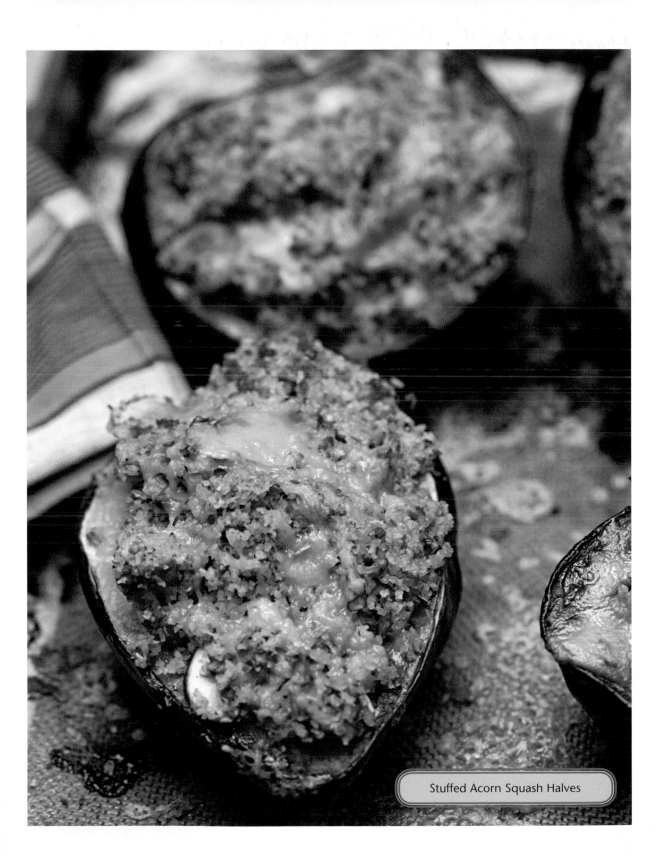

Stuffed Acorn Squash Halves

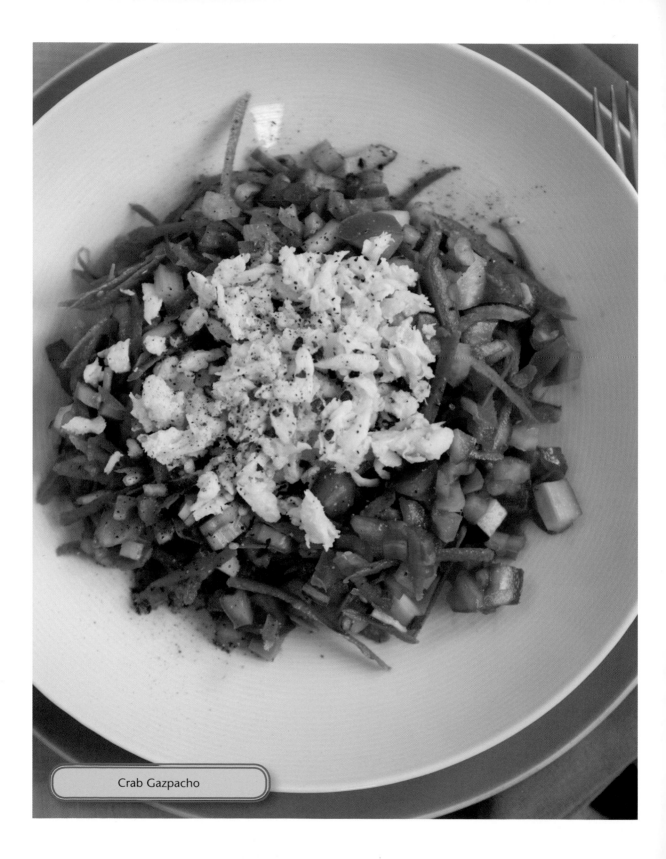

Crab Gazpacho

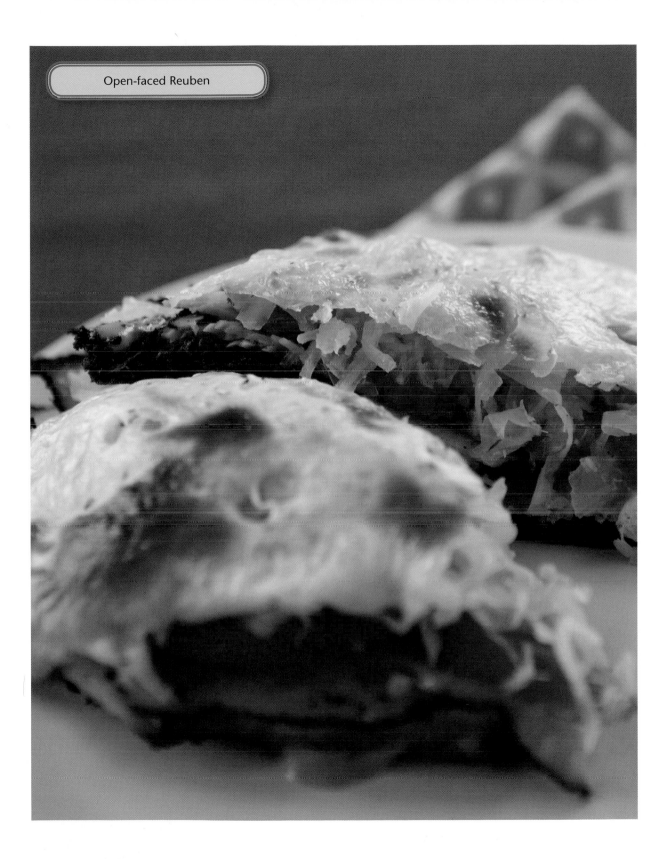

Open-faced Reuben

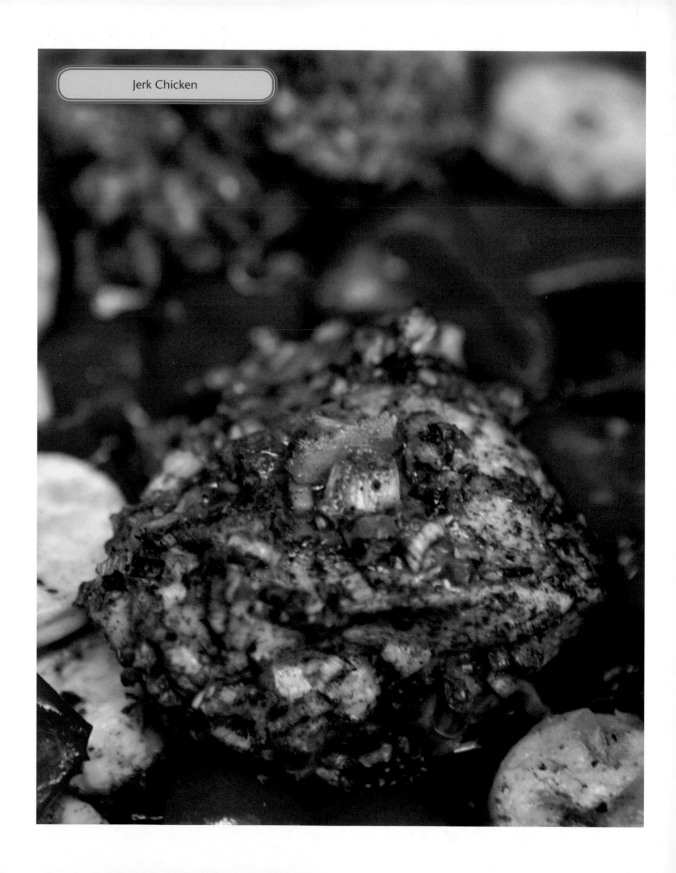

Jerk Chicken

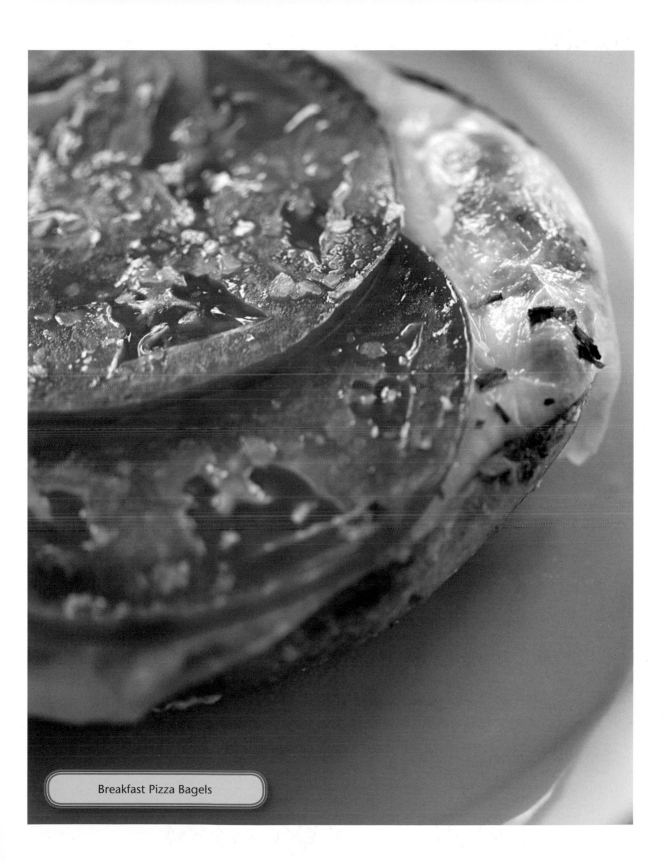

Breakfast Pizza Bagels

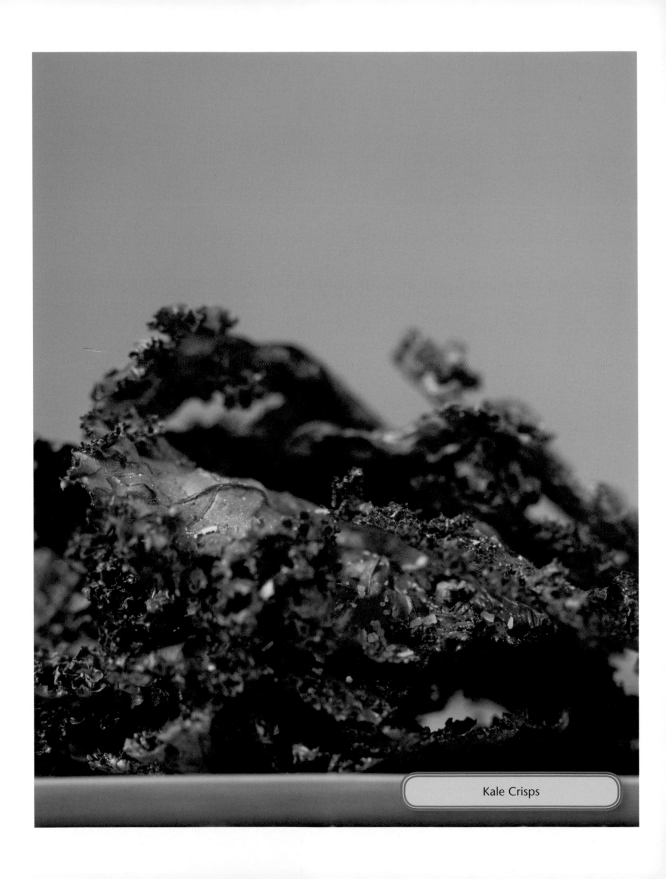

Kale Crisps

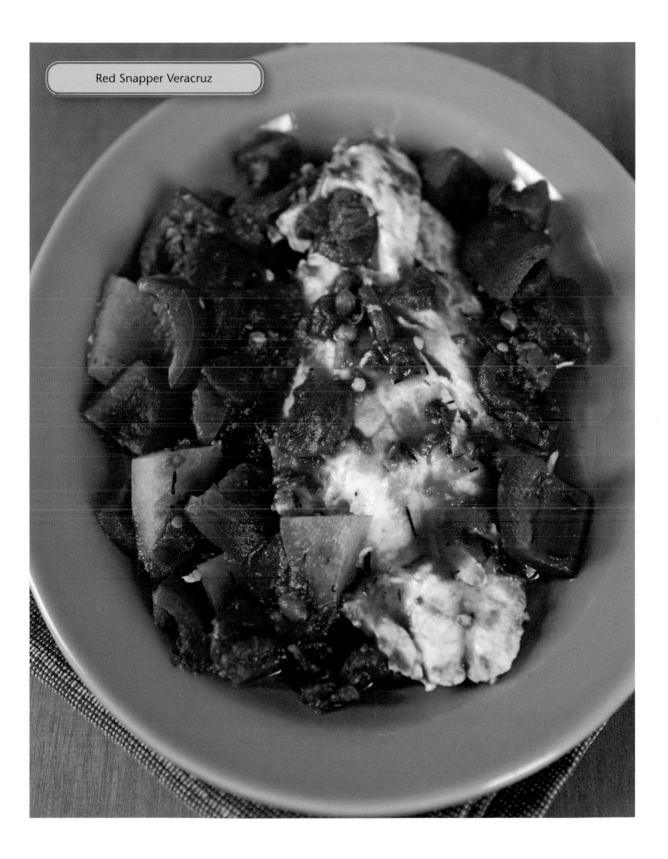

Red Snapper Veracruz

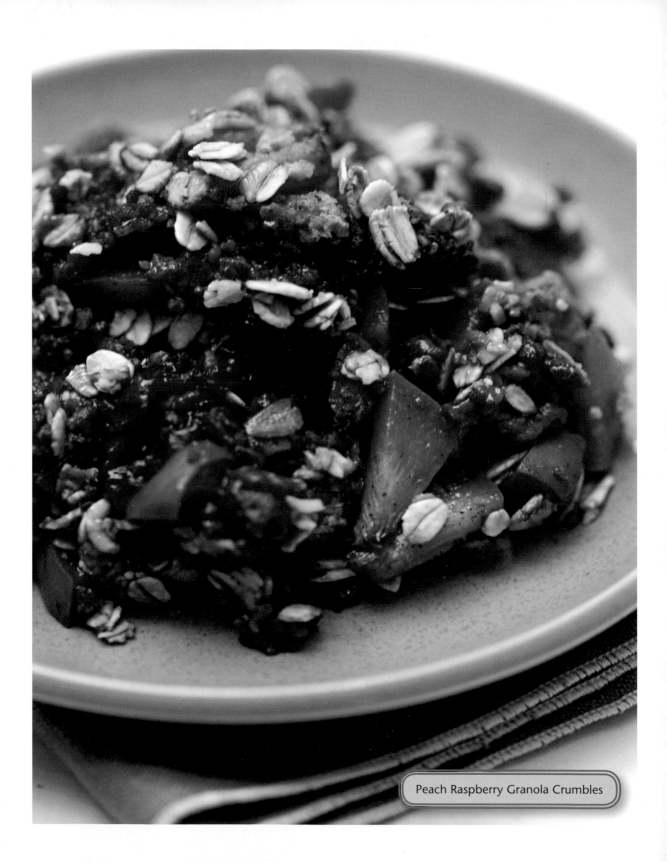

Peach Raspberry Granola Crumbles

Oven-fried Pork Chops

Few pork dishes are more delectable than pan-fried pork chops, but who needs all that fat? An alternative is oven-frying, in which you bread the chops with nutritious wholemeal breadcrumbs and use just a few sprays of non-stick cooking spray to impart a fried feel. Then bake and voilà . . . *I defy anyone to tell the difference.*

INGREDIENTS

4 centre-cut boneless pork loin chops, about 115 g/4 oz each and 1-cm/½-inch thick

200 g/7 oz dried wholemeal breadcrumbs

1 tablespoon Italian seasoning blend

350 ml/12 fl oz reduced-fat buttermilk

Non-stick cooking spray

DIRECTIONS

1. Position a shelf in the centre of the oven and preheat to Gas Mark 6/200°C/fan oven 180°C.

2. Trim any excess fat from the edges of the pork chops. Mix the breadcrumbs and seasoning blend in a shallow bowl. Pour the buttermilk into a second shallow bowl.

3. Spray a large baking tin with non-stick cooking spray. Dip one pork chop into the buttermilk, coating thoroughly on both sides. Hold the pork chop over the bowl for a moment to drain off any excess buttermilk. Put it in the breadcrumbs; press these on to the chop on both sides. Transfer to the baking tray. Repeat with the 3 remaining pork chops.

4. Spray the tops of the pork chops with non-stick cooking spray. Bake until browned and cooked through, about 15 minutes.

YIELD: 4 servings

Slow-cooker Pulled Pork

Attention, barbecue lovers! That should be just about everyone. No longer is the barbecue off limits whilst you're shedding pounds. This has all the bold, meaty, tangy flavour you crave in a plate of great barbecued pork.

INGREDIENTS

1 large white onion, peeled and chopped

250 ml/8 fl oz sugar-free, no-calorie barbecue sauce

1 tablespoon chilli powder

900 g/2 lb boneless centre-cut pork loin, trimmed of all surface fat

DIRECTIONS

1. Mix the onion, barbecue sauce and chilli powder in a 5- to 6-litre/ 8½- to 10-pint slow cooker. Nestle the pork loin in the sauce.

2. Cover and cook on low for 8 to 10 hours, until the pork is falling-apart tender. Shred the meat, using forks. Stir well to combine with the sauce.

YIELD: 8 servings

> **TIPS:** The pulled pork freezes very well. Take the remaining servings and divide into individual containers for freezing so you can have a pulled pork lunch from the microwave anytime.

Lamb and Sweet Potato Stew

Preparing this tasty lamb stew is easy and not especially time consuming. Once it's on the table, you'll have a one-pot meal loaded with nutrition. Make sure you get your lamb well trimmed of all the white fat, because lamb can be on the fatty side.

INGREDIENTS

900 g/2 lb boneless leg of lamb, cut into 1-cm/½-inch pieces

900 g/2 lb sweet potatoes, peeled and cut into thin spears

225 g/8 oz thinly sliced white button mushrooms

4 large shallots, peeled and halved

8 whole garlic cloves, peeled

250 ml/8 fl oz fat-free, low-sodium chicken stock

1 tablespoon sugar-free orange marmalade

2 teaspoons chopped fresh rosemary leaves or 1 teaspoon dried rosemary, crushed

½ teaspoon salt

½ teaspoon black pepper

DIRECTIONS

1. Place all the ingredients in a large pan on the hob or in a 5- to 6-litre/8½- to 10-pint slow cooker and stir until well combined.

2. If using a pan, cover and bring to a simmer, then reduce the heat to low and cook until the meat and potatoes are tender, for about 2½ hours. If using a slow cooker, cover and cook on low for 8 to 10 hours.

YIELD: 8 servings

> **TIP:** Ask the butcher to cube the meat from a boneless leg of lamb for you if not available in the fresh meat section in your supermarket. This will make life so much easier!

Polynesian Grilled Beef

Ready for a big, beefy taste? Try this over-the-top recipe. This beef isn't tender like filet mignon. However, after a long bath in pineapple, soy sauce, spring onions, ginger and garlic, even this rather tough slab of beef turns out a tender close second to a filet. Marinades like this one also add flavour to steak. Then get barbecueing! Can't you just hear the sizzle and smell that unmistakable grilled aroma?

INGREDIENTS

165 g/5¾ oz fresh pineapple, finely chopped

125 ml/4 fl oz light soy sauce

2 medium spring onions, thinly sliced

1 medium garlic clove, finely chopped or 1 teaspoon ready-prepared finely chopped garlic

1 tablespoon peeled, finely chopped, fresh root ginger or ready-prepared, finely chopped root ginger

1 teaspoon Truvia

Non-stick cooking spray

680 g/1 lb 8 oz top round beef

DIRECTIONS

1. Stir the pineapple, soy sauce, spring onions, garlic, ginger and Truvia in a medium bowl. Set the beef in a shallow ovenproof dish and pour the pineapple mixture over the meat. Cover and refrigerate for at least 6 hours or overnight, turning occasionally.

2. Spray the barbecue rack or grill rack with cooking spray. Prepare the barbecue for direct, high-heat cooking or heat the grill pan under a medium-high preheated grill. Place the meat on the barbecue rack directly over the heat or in the grill pan. Cook, basting often with the remaining marinade and fruit in the ovenproof dish, until cooked the way you like it – about 12 minutes for medium rare, about 14 minutes for medium. Transfer to a carving board and let stand for 5 minutes. Cut the beef diagonally across grain into thin slices.

YIELD: 6 servings

TIP: To find the grain of the beef for carving it properly, run your fingers across its surface. You'll see the grain open up, like the grain of wood. For the most tender cuts, slice the beef diagonally across that grain.

Beef Barley Soup

I love this soup, especially on wintry nights. It's so easy to make. All you have to do is toss the ingredients in a saucepan. The hard part is waiting two hours until it's ready! You'll be serving up a filling bowl of nutrition, too. Barley is one of the highest fibre grains you can eat, and fibre is a fat-burner.

INGREDIENTS

- 350 g/12 oz stewing steak, trimmed and cut into 1-cm/½-inch pieces
- 1.4 litres/2¼ pints fat-free beef stock
- 175 g/6 oz white button mushrooms, thinly sliced
- 1 medium white onion, chopped
- 1 large carrot, thinly sliced
- 2 celery sticks, thinly sliced
- 125 g/4½ oz barley
- 1 tablespoon fresh thyme leaves or 1½ teaspoons dried thyme
- ½ teaspoon salt
- ½ teaspoon ground black pepper
- 1 bay leaf
- Several dashes Tabasco sauce, optional

DIRECTIONS

1. Combine the beef, stock, mushrooms, onion, carrot, celery, barley, thyme, salt, pepper and bay leaf in a large saucepan and bring to a full simmer over a medium-high heat, stirring occasionally.

2. Cover, reduce the heat to low and simmer slowly until the beef is tender, for about 2 hours, stirring once in a while. Discard the bay leaf and stir in Tabasco sauce, if using, before serving.

YIELD: 4 servings

Jerk Chicken

A Jamaica-derived dish, true jerk chicken takes hours of slow cooking, but you can get a hint of the flavour, and a great meal, by rubbing the chicken with the spices listed here. Note that the recipe includes plantains, which are close cousins to bananas, and a nutrition-packed alternative to rice and other starches. About 150 g/5½ oz of plantain supplies nearly half your daily vitamin C requirement, more than a third of the vitamin A, and provides three grams of fibre.

INGREDIENTS

- 4 medium spring onions, finely chopped
- 1 small fresh jalapeño pepper, deseeded and finely chopped
- 1 tablespoon apple-cider vinegar
- 2 teaspoons peeled, finely chopped, fresh root ginger or ready-prepared, finely chopped root ginger
- 1 medium garlic clove, finely chopped, or 1 teaspoon ready-prepared finely chopped garlic
- 1 teaspoon olive oil
- 1 teaspoon Truvia
- ½ teaspoon ground allspice
- ½ teaspoon ground coriander
- ½ teaspoon dried thyme
- ½ teaspoon ground cinnamon
- ½ teaspoon salt
- ½ teaspoon ground black pepper
- 3 bone-in skinless chicken breasts, about 225 g/8 oz each and cut in half across
- 1 plantain, peeled and sliced
- 1 medium red pepper, deseeded and coarsely chopped

DIRECTIONS

1. Mix the spring onions, jalapeño, vinegar, ginger, garlic, oil, Truvia, mixed spice, coriander, thyme, cinnamon, salt and pepper in a small bowl.

(continued on next page)

Jerk Chicken (*cont.*)

2. Place the chicken in a 23- x 33-cm/9- x 13-inch ovenproof dish and use a rubber palette knife to spread the jerk marinade over the pieces. Sprinkle the plantain and pepper pieces around the dish. Cover with kitchen foil and refrigerate for at least 2 hours or up to 6 hours.

3. Position a shelf in the centre of the oven and preheat to Gas Mark 5/190°C/fan oven 170°C.

4. Bake, covered, for 15 minutes. Uncover and continue baking until the chicken is cooked through and the plantains are tender, for about 20 more minutes.

YIELD: 4 servings

> **TIPS:** To save time, use 90 ml/3 fl oz cup wet jerk seasoning rub instead of making your own spice blend. Do not use a dry spice blend. You want the wet stuff.
>
> For much more heat and even a more authentic taste, substitute 1 deseeded and finely chopped habanero chilli for the jalapeño.
>
> When working with hot chillies, wear rubber gloves to avoid burns. Failing that, rub your hands thoroughly with olive oil before you wash them to dissolve the chemical that causes the hot burn. Don't touch your eyes, ears, mouth or any sensitive bits with unwashed hands.

Chicken and Apricot Sauté

If your attempts to eat lean and get lean have left you bored with skinless chicken breasts, the Chicken and Apricot Sauté below will be a tasty pleasant surprise, and it is so quick to make. The breasts are sautéed, then doused with a warm apricot sauce that introduces a new dimension to the dish. Amongst fruits, apricots are some of the highest in health-boosting antioxidants.

INGREDIENTS
- 4 boneless skinless chicken breasts, about 115 g/4 oz each
- ½ teaspoon salt
- ½ teaspoon ground black pepper
- 1 tablespoon olive oil
- ½ small red onion, chopped
- 4 medium apricots, stoned and thinly sliced
- 125 ml/4 fl oz fat-free, low-sodium chicken stock
- 2 teaspoons fresh thyme leaves or 1 teaspoon dried thyme
- 2 teaspoons apple-cider vinegar

DIRECTIONS
1. Season the chicken breasts with salt and pepper.
2. Heat ½ tablespoon olive oil in a large frying pan, preferably non-stick. Add the chicken and cook until brown and cooked through, for about 8 minutes, turning once. Transfer the chicken breasts to four serving plates or a serving platter.
3. Add the remaining ½ tablespoon oil to the frying pan. Add the onion and apricot slices and cook, stirring almost constantly, for 2 minutes. Stir in the stock and thyme and bring to a full boil. Boil for 1 minute. Stir in the vinegar, boil for 30 seconds and spoon the sauce over the chicken breasts.

YIELD: 4 servings

TIP: Substitute walnut oil or almond oil for the olive oil, for a subtle change in flavour.

Turkey and Mushroom Sloppy Joes

How's this for luscious and low-fat? Ounce for ounce, turkey breast yields less dietary fat than chicken breast or any cut of the leanest beef. In 115 g/4 oz of turkey breast there is just a single gram of fat but a whopping 26 grams of protein. In these oh-so-delicious American Sloppy Joes, sort of like bolognese on toast, we've taken the fat and calories down a few more notches by replacing some of the meatiness with meaty-tasting mushrooms.

INGREDIENTS

550 g/1 lb 4 oz white button or chestnut mushrooms, thinly sliced

1 tablespoon olive oil

350 g/12 oz lean turkey mince

1 medium white onion, chopped

3 medium garlic cloves, finely chopped, or 1 tablespoon ready-prepared finely chopped garlic

2 tablespoons balsamic vinegar

2 tablespoons Worcestershire sauce

1 tablespoon finely chopped fresh oregano or 1½ teaspoons dried oregano

135 g/4¾ oz tomato purée

2 tablespoons calorie-free barbecue sauce

½ teaspoon salt

½ teaspoon ground black pepper

4 slices wholegrain toast

DIRECTIONS

1. Place the mushrooms in a food processor fitted with the chopping blade. Process until ground to the consistency of minced steak.

2. Heat the oil in a large saucepan over a medium heat. Add the turkey mince and cook, stirring often, until it loses its raw, pink colour, for about 4 minutes.

3. Add mushrooms, onion and garlic. Continue cooking, stirring often, until the onions soften and the mushrooms give off most

of their liquid, for about 3 minutes. Stir in the vinegar, Worcestershire sauce and oregano and simmer for 1 minute.

4. Stir in the tomato purée, barbecue sauce, salt and pepper. Cook, stirring constantly to prevent scorching, until thick, to the point at which the mixture will hold its shape on a spoon, for about 8 minutes. Serve on toast.

YIELD: 4 servings

> **TIP:** It's important to have those mushrooms really finely chopped. If you don't own a food processor, you can put the mushrooms on a chopping board and rock a large knife through them repeatedly, slowly grinding/chopping them to the right consistency. You really have to go at it. Even when you think it's finely chopped, do some more work with the knife, just to be sure.

Stuffed Acorn Squash Halves

Here's a novel, scrumptious way to prepare acorn squash, a treat that earns its keep as a nutrient-rich veggie. A typical serving of acorn squash provides about 40 per cent of the adult daily requirement for vitamin A, as well as contributing B vitamins and some iron and other minerals. It is also a fairly rich source of potassium. This dish makes a tasty complement to just about any meat main dish.

INGREDIENTS

Non-stick cooking spray

2 medium acorn squashes, halved and seeds and membranes removed

140 g/5 oz quick-cooking bulgar

115 g/4 oz reduced-fat turkey sausage meat, crumbled

225 g/8 oz white button or chestnut mushrooms, thinly sliced

1 tablespoon Italian seasoning blend

2 tablespoons sweet chilli sauce

30 g/1 oz low-fat Cheddar cheese, coarsely grated

DIRECTIONS

1. Position a shelf in the centre of the oven and preheat to Gas Mark 4/180°C/fan oven 160°C.

2. Spray a 23- x 33-cm/9- x 13-inch ovenproof dish with non-stick cooking spray. Set the squash halves, cut side down, in the dish. Bake until tender when pierced through the skin with a knife, for about 45 minutes.

3. Meanwhile, put the bulgar in a large heatproof bowl, pour in 350 ml/12 fl oz boiling water, stir, cover and set aside for 30 minutes or until all the water has been absorbed.

4. Spray a large frying pan with the non-stick cooking spray and set over a medium heat. Add the sausage meat and cook, stirring often, until browned, for about 5 minutes.

5. Add the mushrooms and cook, stirring occasionally, until they give off their liquid, for about a further 5 minutes. Stir in the bulgar, seasoning blend and chilli sauce. Stir until uniform.

6. Once the squash halves are tender, use oven gloves or tongs to turn them over without piercing them. Divide the turkey mixture between the halves, filling the cavities. Top each with 1 tablespoon of the cheese. Bake until the cheese has melted and browned a bit, for about 10 minutes. Cool for 5 minutes before serving.

YIELD: 4 servings

TIPS: Substitute crumbled soya sausage, if you wish. Scrub the squash really well. When tender, the skin is edible.

Amaranth Polenta

Polenta is usually made with ground corn, but you can make it with amaranth, too. Amaranth is a wholegrain that offers something processed grains don't: lots of high-quality protein. It's also a natural source of fibre, iron, calcium and phosphorus.

INGREDIENTS

2 teaspoons olive oil

2 medium shallots, peeled, halved and thinly sliced

175 g/6 oz white button or chestnut mushrooms, thinly sliced

350 ml/12 fl oz vegetable stock

200 g/7 oz wholegrain amaranth

1 teaspoon dried thyme

½ teaspoon salt

½ teaspoon black pepper

2 tablespoons finely grated Parmigiano-Reggiano

DIRECTIONS

1. Heat the oil in a medium saucepan over a medium heat. Add the shallots and cook, stirring often, until softened, for about 2 minutes. Add the mushrooms and cook, stirring occasionally, until they give off their liquid and it coats the pan, for about 2 minutes.

2. Stir in the stock, amaranth, thyme, salt and pepper. Raise the heat to medium-high and bring to a full boil. Cover, reduce the heat to low and simmer until thick and polenta-like, for about 30 minutes, stirring several times. Stir in the cheese.

YIELD: 4 servings

> **TIP:** Make sure you use wholegrain, preferably organic, amaranth, not amaranth grits. You can find it at large supermarkets in the organic aisle or at health food shops. It cooks into something like polenta but stickier. And it will firm up if you don't eat it quickly, say, within 10 minutes. So, you can't make it ahead and set it on the back of the hob. Still, it makes a great side dish!

Courgette, Lemon and Parmesan Sauté

The French and the British use the term courgette, which has more to do with its scientific name Curcurbita than its historical heritage. Italians took this tasty veggie and its name, zucchino, with them to America in the early twentieth century. It's so versatile that you can eat it raw, add it to salads, steam it, boil it, bake it, stuff it and more. Here we sauté it. When it comes to nutrition, courgettes are great. About 100 g/3½ oz of sliced courgette is packed with vitamin C and supplies only 16 calories.

INGREDIENTS

2 medium courgettes
Non-stick cooking spray
½ teaspoon salt
Finely grated zest from 1 medium lemon
30 g/1 oz flaked almonds, toasted
3 tablespoons finely grated Parmigiano-Reggiano
½ teaspoon ground black pepper

DIRECTIONS

1. Grate the courgettes through the large holes of a box grater and into a large bowl. Squeeze handfuls of the grated courgette over the sink to remove excess moisture.

2. Spray a large frying pan with non-stick cooking spray and set over a medium heat for 1 minute. Add the courgettes and cook, stirring often, until wilted, for about 2 minutes. Stir in the salt and lemon zest and continue to stir over the heat for 1 minute.

3. Remove the frying pan from the heat. Stir in the almonds and cheese. Top with pepper and serve.

YIELD: 4 servings

> **TIP:** To toast flaked almonds, put them in a dry frying pan over a low heat and cook for about 3 minutes, stirring occasionally. You can sometimes find toasted almonds at the supermarket.

Kale Crisps

All hail, kale crisps! You'll no longer need to worry about satisfying cravings for fattening potato crisps once you've tried these. Crunch a few and you'll never have your hand in a packet of crisps again, or at least I hope not!

INGREDIENTS
450 g/1 lb kale leaves, washed and dried
Non-stick cooking spray
½ teaspoon salt

DIRECTIONS

1. Position shelves in the top and bottom thirds of the oven; preheat to Gas Mark 5/180°C/fan oven 160°C.

2. Cut out the thick centre stalks from the kale leaves and tear the leaves themselves into ragged 7.5-cm/3-inch pieces.

3. Spray two large baking trays with non-stick cooking spray. Lay the leaf pieces on them in a single layer. Spray the leaves lightly with non-stick cooking spray.

4. Set the trays on the two racks. Bake for 15 minutes. Use tongs to turn the leaves over, then reverse the trays top to bottom. Continue baking until crisp, about 15 more minutes. Sprinkle with salt whilst hot.

YIELD: 4 servings

TIP: Make sure the kale leaves are completely dry before you start this recipe.

Three Popcorn Spice Mixes

Popcorn is one of the healthiest snacks around. It's low in calories (about 23 calories per 8 g/¼ oz) and high in fibre. Only when soaked in butter and showered in salt does it become fattening. Because of this, most of us try to eat popcorn plain. However, there are other ways to enjoy it; here's how to spice up your popcorn experience.

INGREDIENTS

Parmesan and Herb

30 g/1 oz fresh Parmigiano-Reggiano cheese, finely grated
½ teaspoon dried thyme
½ teaspoon dried oregano
½ teaspoon dried basil
½ teaspoon salt
½ teaspoon ground black pepper

Curried Cheddar

40 g/1½ oz low-fat Cheddar cheese, finely grated
½ teaspoon curry powder
½ teaspoon onion powder
½ teaspoon salt
¼ teaspoon garlic powder

Cajun Spice

2 teaspoons mild paprika
½ teaspoon dried thyme
½ teaspoon onion powder
½ teaspoon celery seeds
½ teaspoon salt
¼ teaspoon garlic powder
¼ teaspoon cayenne

(continued on next page)

Three Popcorn Spice Mixes (*cont.*)

DIRECTIONS

To make spiced popcorn, put 30 g/1 oz popped popcorn in a large bowl and spray lightly with non-stick cooking spray. Mix one of the spice blends in a small bowl and sprinkle over the popcorn. Toss well.

YIELD: 4 servings

> **TIP:** Use fresh Parmigiano-Reggiano for recipes and grate it yourself with the small holes of a box grater or a microplane. The ready-grated Parmesan in packets on sale in supermarkets is often made with lots of oils and chemical fillers. Better to buy a chunk of this cheese and keep it tightly wrapped in the fridge until you need it.

Stuffed Figs

Here's a fig deal for you: scrumptiously stuffed figs that taste every bit as yummy as chocolate sweeties. Figs are loaded with magnesium, calcium, potassium, even a little protein and zinc. The biggest nutrition bonanza in this fruit is its fibre. For people taking laxatives, include more figs in your diet, and you won't need them.

INGREDIENTS
    4 large figs
    60 g/2¼ oz soft, fresh goat's cheese (chèvre)
    ¼ teaspoon ground black pepper
    4 walnut halves
    60 ml/2 fl oz sugar-free chocolate sauce

DIRECTIONS
Split each fig from the stalk down without cutting all the way through to the base. Open the slit a bit and spread 15 g/½ oz goat's cheese inside the fig. Sprinkle the cheese with black pepper and place a walnut half in each fig. Set the figs on serving plates and drizzle each with 1 tablespoon chocolate sauce.

YIELD: 4 servings

> **TIP:** For more flavour, toast the walnut halves in a dry frying pan for a couple of minutes and cool completely before using. Sugar-free chocolate sauces vary in flavour and goodness; you might need to experiment with a few to find the best one.

Peach Raspberry Granola Crumbles

This recipe is a take on traditional fruit crumble, only healthier and virtually fat free. It's even okay to serve it for breakfast.

INGREDIENTS

Non-stick cooking spray
1 large peach, stoned and chopped
185 g/6½ oz raspberries
2 tablespoons wholemeal breadcrumbs
2 teaspoons Truvia
½ teaspoon ground cinnamon
125 g/4½ oz low-fat granola

DIRECTIONS

1. Position a shelf in the centre of the oven and preheat to Gas Mark 4/180°C/fan oven 160°C.

2. Spray 4 holes in a bun tin with non-stick cooking spray. Mix the peaches, raspberries, breadcrumbs, Truvia and cinnamon in a bowl; divide among the holes in the tin. Top each with a quarter of the granola.

3. Bake until bubbling and hot, for about 30 minutes. Cool for 5 minutes in the tin before scooping into bowls.

YIELD: 4 servings

TIP: The granola should be fairly plain, without added dried fruit such as raisins, for example. You don't want any complicated flavours to compete with the peaches and raspberries.

Baked Bananas

Bananas alone make a great dessert, but wait until you liven them up like this! Yummy and full of nutrition, they're a great way to get your fat-burning probiotics in.

INGREDIENTS

Non-stick cooking spray

4 large bananas, peeled

80 g/2¾ oz no-added-sugar apricot jam or all-fruit spread

1 teaspoon vanilla essence

¼ teaspoon ground cinnamon

115 g/4 oz sugar-free, low-fat vanilla yoghurt or Greek yoghurt

DIRECTIONS

1. Position a shelf in the centre of the oven and preheat to Gas Mark 6/200°C/fan oven 180°C.

2. Lightly spray the inside of a small baking tin with non-stick cooking spray. Set the bananas in the tin. Spread the jam over the bananas and sprinkle with the vanilla and cinnamon. Cover the ovenproof dish with kitchen foil and bake for 20 minutes. Scoop the bananas and sauce on to plates and top each serving with 2 tablespoons yoghurt.

YIELD: 4 servings

TIP: Make sure that the foil is sealed tightly. You can also use peach all-fruit spread instead, or even a sugar-free fig spread.

Grilled Pineapple with Vanilla Ricotta and Pistachios

Think of this dessert as a pineapple sundae, because that's what it tastes like. I don't want to spoil that image for you, but the doctor in me does have to add something about how healthy this recipe is: full of protein, calcium, fibre and natural enzymes.

INGREDIENTS

Non-stick cooking spray

1 large pineapple, peeled, cored, and chopped into 2.5-cm/ 1-inch-thick spears

450 g/1 lb low-fat ricotta cheese

2 teaspoons Truvia

2 teaspoons vanilla extract

60 g/2¼ oz shelled pistachios, chopped

DIRECTIONS

1. Spray a barbecue rack or a grill pan with non-stick cooking spray. Prepare the barbecue for direct, high-heat cooking, or heat the grill pan under a medium-high preheated grill, until smoking.

2. Set the pineapple spears on the barbecue rack directly over the heat or in the grill pan. Grill until marked and hot, for about 4 minutes, turning once. Divide the spears between four plates.

3. Mix the ricotta, Truvia and vanilla in a small bowl. Dollop a quarter on top of the grilled pineapple on each plate. Sprinkle with chopped pistachios.

YIELD: 4 servings

TIP: You can often find peeled, cored pineapple in the chilled section of the produce aisles, often sealed in a plastic container. Simply use the pineapple rings rather than the spears.

17 Sample Cycle 3 Menus

Here are examples of how to build menus using the preceding recipes whilst on the Achieve Cycle. You can follow these menus exactly or create your own.

Day 1

Breakfast

☐ 1 serving *Better Migas*

☐ ½ grapefruit or other fresh fruit

☐ 1 cup green tea

Lunch

☐ 1 serving *Spinach Mushroom Salad with Warm Bacon Dressing*

☐ 1 serving fresh fruit

☐ 1 cup green tea

Dinner

☐ 1 serving *Slow-cooker Pulled Pork*

☐ 30-55 g/1-2 oz tossed mixed salad with 2 tablespoons fat-free dressing

☐ 1 cup green tea

Snacks

☐ 1 probiotic, dairy or dairy-substitute serving

☐ 1 frozen fruit ice lolly

Day 2

Breakfast

- ☐ 40 g/1½ oz high-fibre cereal, such as bran flakes
- ☐ 250 ml/8 fl oz low-fat or soya milk or other dairy substitute
- ☐ 125 g/4½ oz fresh berries
- ☐ 1 cup green tea

Lunch

- ☐ 1 serving *White Bean and Oat Burgers*
- ☐ 10 baby carrots
- ☐ 1 cup green tea

Dinner

- ☐ 1 serving *Jerk Chicken*
- ☐ Steamed vegetables such as asparagus, runner beans, broccoli or cauliflower
- ☐ 1 cup green tea

Snacks

- ☐ 1 serving *Stuffed Figs*
- ☐ 1 Skinny Cow Skinny Sticks ice cream lolly

Day 3

Breakfast

☐ 1 serving *Banana Chocolate Smoothie*

☐ 1 slice wholegrain toast

☐ 1 cup green tea

Lunch

☐ 1 serving *Crab Gazpacho*

☐ 1 cup green tea

Dinner

☐ 1 serving *Lamb and Sweet Potato Stew*

☐ 1 cup green tea

Snacks

☐ 1 serving *Baked Bananas*

☐ 2nd probiotic, dairy or dairy-substitute serving

Day 4

Breakfast

☐ 1 *Dr Mike's Power Cookie*

☐ 250 ml/8 fl oz low-fat or soya milk or other dairy substitute

☐ 125 g/4½ oz fresh berries

☐ 1 cup green tea

Lunch

☐ 1 serving *Prawn Soba Noodle Salad*

☐ 1 medium apple or pear

☐ 1 cup green tea

Dinner

☐ 1 bowl *Beef Barley Soup*

☐ 1 cup green tea

Snacks

☐ 2nd probiotic, dairy or dairy-substitute serving

☐ *Kale Crisps*

Day 5

Breakfast

☐ 2 scrambled eggs

☐ 1 serving *Slow-cooker Brown Rice Congee*

☐ 125 g/4½ oz fresh berries

☐ 1 cup green tea

Lunch

☐ 1 serving *Easy Cioppino*

☐ 1 fresh pear

☐ 1 cup green tea

Dinner

☐ 1 serving *Oven-fried Pork Chops*

☐ Steamed broccoli

☐ 30-55 g/1-2 oz tossed mixed salad with 2 tablespoons fat-free dressing

☐ 1 cup green tea

Snacks

☐ Probiotic, dairy or dairy-substitute serving

☐ 1 100-calorie chocolate-flavoured ice lolly

NOTES

Day 6

Breakfast

☐ 225 g/8 oz sugar-free, fruit-flavoured yoghurt

☐ 60 g/2¼ oz low-fat granola

☐ 1 piece fresh fruit (i.e., 1 peach, ¼ cantaloupe, ½ grapefruit or 1 orange)

☐ 1 cup green tea

Lunch

☐ 1 serving *Crab Cakes*

☐ Medium jacket potato with 1 tablespoon fat-free soured cream; or 100 g cooked brown basmati rice

☐ 1 medium apple

☐ 1 cup green tea

Dinner

☐ 1 serving *Polynesian Grilled Beef*

☐ Yellow squash, steamed

☐ 1 cup green tea

Snack

☐ 2nd probiotic, dairy or dairy-substitute serving

☐ 1 frozen fruit ice lolly

Day 7

Breakfast

☐ 1 serving *Grilled Pineapple with Vanilla Ricotta and Pistachios*

☐ 1 cup green tea

Lunch

☐ 1 serving *Tex-Mex Millet Salad*

☐ 1 cup green tea

Dinner

☐ 1 serving *Roasted Trout Almandine*

☐ Steamed vegetables

☐ 30-55 g/1-2 oz tossed mixed salad with 2 tablespoons reduced-fat dressing

☐ 1 cup green tea

Snacks

☐ 175 g/6 oz natural or sugar-free, fruit-flavoured yoghurt

☐ 1 serving fresh fruit, in season

Day 8

Breakfast

- ☐ 1 *Dr Mike's Power Cookie*
- ☐ 1 banana, sliced
- ☐ 250 ml/8 fl oz skimmed milk
- ☐ 1 cup green tea

Lunch

- ☐ 1 serving *Brie and Mango Quesadilla*
- ☐ Spinach, steamed
- ☐ 1 cup green tea

Dinner

- ☐ 1 serving *Grilled Miso-glazed Salmon*
- ☐ 1 serving *Stuffed Acorn Squash Halves*
- ☐ 1 cup green tea

Snacks

- ☐ 1 probiotic, dairy or dairy-substitute serving
- ☐ 1 frozen fruit ice lolly

Day 9

Breakfast

☐ 1 serving *Breakfast Pizza Bagels*

☐ 125 g/4½ oz fresh berries

☐ 1 cup green tea

Lunch

☐ 1 serving *Open-faced Reuben*

☐ 1 cup green tea

Dinner

☐ 1 serving *Chicken and Apricot Sauté*

☐ Steamed vegetables such as asparagus, runner beans, broccoli or cauliflower

☐ 1 cup green tea

Snacks

☐ *Kale Crisps*

☐ 1 Skinny Cow Skinny Stick ice-cream lolly

NOTES

Breakfast

- ☐ 115 g/4 oz cooked porridge
- ☐ ½ grapefruit
- ☐ 1 cup green tea

Lunch

- ☐ 1 serving *Crab Gazpacho*
- ☐ 1 cup green tea

Dinner

- ☐ 1 serving *Turkey and Mushroom Sloppy Joes*
- ☐ 30-55 g/1-2 oz tossed mixed salad with 2 tablespoons reduced-fat dressing
- ☐ 1 cup green tea

Snacks

- ☐ 2nd fruit serving
- ☐ 2nd probiotic, dairy or dairy-substitute serving

Day 11

Breakfast

☐ 1 serving *Better Migas*

☐ 1 medium apple or pear

☐ 1 cup green tea

Lunch

☐ 1 serving *Crab Cakes*

☐ 30-55 g/1-2 oz tossed mixed salad with 2 tablespoons reduced-fat dressing

☐ 1 cup green tea

Dinner

☐ 1 serving *Red Snapper Veracruz*

☐ 1 serving *Peach Raspberry Granola Crumbles*

☐ 1 cup green tea

Snacks

☐ 1 serving *Popcorn Spice Mix*

☐ 2nd probiotic, dairy or dairy-substitute serving

Day 12

Breakfast

☐ 4 scrambled egg whites

☐ 1 rasher back bacon

☐ 165 g/5¾ oz diced melon

☐ 1 cup green tea

Lunch

☐ 1 serving *White Bean and Oat Burger*

☐ 1 fresh pear or other fruit in season

☐ 1 cup green tea

Dinner

☐ 1 serving *Arroz con Poussins*

☐ 1 cup green tea

Snacks

☐ Probiotic, dairy or dairy-substitute serving

☐ 1 100-calorie chocolate-flavoured ice lolly

Day 13

Breakfast

- ☐ 175 g/6 oz sugar-free, fruit-flavoured yoghurt
- ☐ 1 piece fresh fruit (i.e, 1 peach, ¼ cantaloupe, ½ grapefruit or 1 orange)
- ☐ 1 cup green tea

Lunch

- ☐ 1 serving *Open-faced Reuben*
- ☐ 1 medium apple
- ☐ 1 cup green tea

Dinner

- ☐ 115-175 g/4-6 oz baked chicken breast
- ☐ 1 serving *Courgette, Lemon and Parmesan Sauté*
- ☐ 1 cup green tea

Snack

- ☐ 2nd probiotic, dairy or-dairy substitute serving
- ☐ 1 serving *Stuffed Figs*

Day 14

Breakfast

☐ 2 scrambled eggs

☐ 1 serving *Slow-cooker Brown Rice Congee*

☐ 165 g/5¾ oz pineapple chunks, fresh or canned in their own juice

☐ 1 cup green tea

Lunch

☐ 1 serving *Brie and Mango Quesadilla*

☐ 30-55 g/1-2 oz tossed mixed salad with 2 tablespoons reduced-fat dressing

☐ 1 cup green tea

Dinner

☐ 1 serving *Slow-cooker Pulled Pork*

☐ 100 g/3½ oz shredded cabbage tossed with low-fat coleslaw dressing

☐ 1 cup green tea

Snack

☐ 2nd probiotic, dairy or dairy-substitute serving

☐ 1 medium orange

Day 15

Breakfast

☐ 1 serving *Banana Chocolate Smoothie*

☐ 1 cup green tea

Lunch

☐ 1 serving *Tex-Mex Millet Salad*

☐ 125 g/4½ oz fresh berries

☐ 1 cup green tea

Dinner

☐ 1 serving *Prawn Vindaloo*

☐ 30-55 g/1-2 oz tossed mixed salad with 2 tablespoons reduced-fat dressing

☐ 1 cup green tea

Snacks

☐ 1 probiotic, dairy or dairy-substitute serving

☐ 1 frozen fruit ice lolly

NOTES

NOTES

Breakfast

☐ 40 g/1½ oz high-fibre cereal, such as bran flakes

☐ 250 ml/8 fl oz low-fat or soya milk or other dairy substitute

☐ 1 banana, sliced

☐ 1 cup green tea

Lunch

☐ 1 serving *Spinach Mushroom Salad with Warm Bacon Dressing*

☐ 1 cup green tea

Dinner

☐ 1 serving *Jerk Chicken*

☐ Steamed vegetables such as asparagus, runner beans, broccoli or cauliflower

☐ 1 cup green tea

Snacks

☐ 2nd fruit serving

☐ 1 Skinny Cow Skinny Stick ice-cream lolly

Day 17

Breakfast

☐ 175 g/6 oz non-fat Greek yoghurt mixed with 1 tablespoon sugar-free fruit jam

☐ 125 g/4½ oz fresh berries

☐ 1 cup green tea

Lunch

☐ 1 serving *Crab Gazpacho*

☐ 1 cup green tea

Dinner

☐ 1 serving *Polynesian Grilled Beef*

☐ 1 medium jacket potato with 1 tablespoon reduced-fat soured cream or Greek yoghurt

☐ 30-55 g/1-2 oz tossed mixed salad with 1 tablespoon oil mixed with 2 tablespoons vinegar

☐ 1 cup green tea

Snacks

☐ 2nd fruit serving

☐ 1 fat-free pudding cup

About Cycle 4: Arrive

After you have reached your goal weight by using Cycles 1 through 3 as directed, you graduate to Cycle 4: Arrive. This is the maintenance cycle of the 17 Day Diet. You fought the battle of the bulge and won. This is a huge, important accomplishment, something many people fail to do. Now, the important thing is that you stay at this weight.

Here's how you do that.

Enjoy yourself on the weekend. Yes, you can splurge on the weekends, if you wish. Let's face it: weekends have never been good for diets. You get a promotion on Friday, so you eat. Or you snuggle up to watch a film on Friday or Saturday, and you eat. Or you go out to a party, and you eat. The problem is, from 6.00 p.m. on Friday until bedtime on Sunday, your life changes. Your schedule is looser, allowing for more snacking. Then there are the social commitments. Dinners out, birthday shindigs, Sunday brunch – they can do you in. It seems like you need thick layers of duct tape on your mouth to prevent gorging.

Taking weekends off allows you to splurge a bit, making it easier to get back on track on Monday. Most people can be pretty good from Monday to Thursday, choosing meals carefully, getting in some exercise and seeing decent results on the scales. The Arrive Cycle capitalises on these normal rhythms of life and builds a *livable* maintenance plan around them.

Besides rapid weight loss, this is the feature of the 17 Day Diet everyone loves. Of course, come Monday morning, you simply minimise any overindulgent damage by getting back on one of the cycles.

Use your favourite cycle, and all your favourite recipes from this cookbook, during the week. On weekdays, stay strict and use your favourite cycle to control your weight. I'm giving you the best diet present you can have. You still eat a calorie-controlled diet during the week, then, on weekends, have what you like. You take off plenty of pounds, and you keep the weight off because you never get bored using my weekend principle.

The Arrive Cycle is metabolically strategic, too. You can control your weight efficiently because you're shocking your metabolism back into action. Why? Because you're following 5 days of controlled eating, followed by 2 days of increased calories. By adding calories to your meals with beefburgers, bread, ice cream, wine, cheesecake, you name it, you're speeding up your metabolism. Then, when your metabolism is roaring like a boiler, you get back to your diet on Monday, burning calories faster than ever. Basically, the Arrive Cycle keeps your metabolism guessing, so it never has a chance to go into hibernation. Since your metabolism is now well trained due to better eating habits and digestive health, a few cheat treats on the weekend will not have an adverse affect.

The Arrive Cycle is not a free-for-all, though. You're allowed some of your favourite foods in moderation. For example, Friday night: a meal with a cocktail or two at your favourite restaurant, Saturday a slice or two of pizza for lunch or dinner, plus one dessert, and Sunday a breakfast of pancakes with maple syrup.

A good rule of thumb to follow whilst stabilising your weight is to enjoy no more than one to three favourite meals each weekend. I call this *strategic cheating*. It works wonders for keeping weight off, and you'll love the freedom.

As a parting shot, let me say that millions of people have lost weight rapidly and safely on the 17 Day Diet. Now with *The 17 Day Diet Workbook* and *The 17 Day Cookbook*, you have more tools than ever to stick with this remarkably effective programme.

What matters to me now is that you use the cookbook to help you arrive at your goal sooner rather than later. Try as many recipes as you can, pick your favourites, enjoy and start loving your new, trimmer, shapelier physique.

Cheers . . . see you at your goal!

INDEX